From: Dorothy Dix
Jan 26th 2004

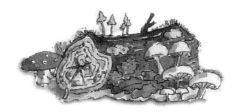

*HEALTH AND HEALING
THE NATURAL WAY*

THE HEALTHY
ENVIRONMENT

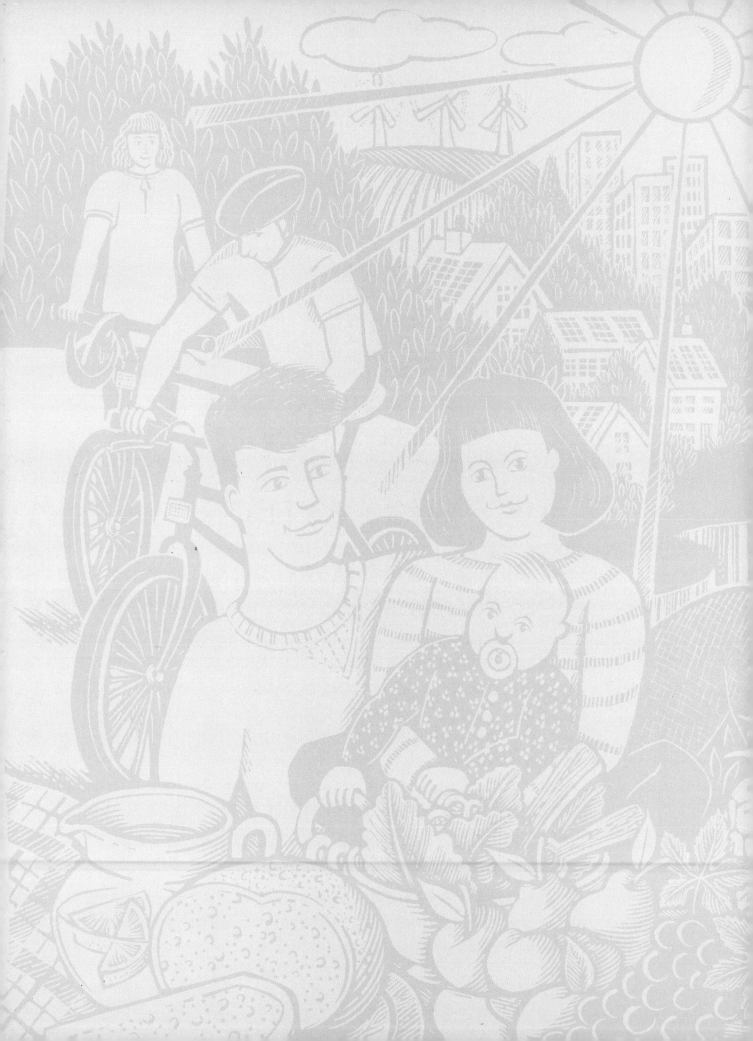

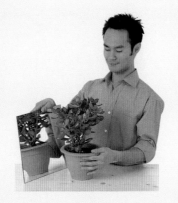

HEALTH AND HEALING
THE NATURAL WAY

THE HEALTHY ENVIRONMENT

Reader's
Digest

PUBLISHED BY

THE READER'S DIGEST ASSOCIATION, INC.

PLEASANTVILLE, NEW YORK / MONTREAL

THE HEALTHY ENVIRONMENT
Produced by
Carroll & Brown Limited, London

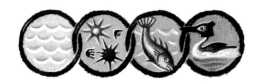

CARROLL & BROWN

Publishing Director Denis Kennedy
Art Director Chrissie Lloyd

Managing Editors Sandra Rigby, Rachel Aris
Managing Art Editor Tracy Timson

Editors Denise Alexander, Caroline Uzielli

Art Editor Sandra Brooke
Designers Julie Bennett, Evie Loizides, Vimit Punater

Photographers Jules Selmes, David Murray

Production Wendy Rogers, Clair Reynolds

Computer Management John Clifford, Elisa Merino,
Paul Stradling

Library of Congress Cataloging in Publication Data

The healthy environment
    p. cm. — (Health and healing the natural way)
    ISBN 0-7621-0283-7
    1. Environmental health.
    I. Reader's Digest Association. II. Series.

RA565 .H397 2001
613—dc21
                                        00-020377

The information in this book is for reference only;
it is not intended as a substitute for a doctor's diagnosis and care.
The editors urge anyone with continuing medical problems
or symptoms to consult a doctor.

CONSULTANT

Dr. Paul Harrison
*Head of Environmental Toxicology, Institute for
Environment and Health, University of Leicester*

CONTRIBUTORS

Tim Brown
*National Society for Clean Air and Environmental
Protection*
Ian MacArthur, Howard Price
Chartered Institute of Environmental Health
John Fawell
Water Research Centre
Sue Stolton
Equilibrium Consultancy
Hugh MacGrillen
London Hazards Centre
Sue Dibb
The Food Commission
Suzy Chiazzari
Holistic Interior Design and Colour Consultant
Richard Emerson
Medical Health Writer
Sue Taylor
London School of Health and Tropical Medicine
Jake Ferguson
Camden Council, Environment and Health Coordinator
Matthew Gaines
Formerly of National Radiological Protection Board

READER'S DIGEST PROJECT STAFF

Series Editor Gayla Visalli
Editorial Director, Health & Medicine Wayne Kalyn
Associate Designer Jennifer R. Tokarski
Production Technology Manager Douglas A. Croll
Editorial Manager Christine R. Guido

READER'S DIGEST ILLUSTRATED REFERENCE BOOKS, U.S.

Editor-in-Chief Christopher Cavanaugh
Art Director Joan Mazzeo
Operations Manager William J. Cassidy

Address any comments about *The Healthy Environment* to
Reader's Digest, Editor-in-Chief, U.S. Illustrated Reference Books,
Reader's Digest Rd., Pleasantville, NY 10570

THE HEALTHY ENVIRONMENT

More and more people today are choosing to take greater responsibility for their own health care rather than relying on a doctor to step in with a cure when something goes wrong. We now recognize that we can influence our health by making improvements in lifestyle—for example, eating better, getting more exercise, and reducing stress. People are also becoming increasingly aware that there are other healing methods—some of them new, others ancient—that can help prevent illness or be used as a complement to orthodox medicine.

The series *Health and Healing the Natural Way* can help you to make your own health choices by giving you clear, comprehensive, straightforward, and encouraging information and advice about methods of improving your health. The series explains the many different natural therapies that are now available, including aromatherapy, herbalism, acupressure, and a number of others, and the circumstances in which they may be of benefit when used in conjunction with conventional medicine.

THE HEALTHY ENVIRONMENT explains exactly what health risks we face today—from pollution in the air we breathe, the water we drink, and the food we eat to radiation from the sun and cellular phones—and what steps we can take to minimize them. Drawing on the expertise of researchers and occupational health and safety advisers, the book examines the evidence for the dangers posed by particular hazards and shows how our own actions can have a major impact on improving conditions. The surprising extent to which the home and office can threaten health is explored—from the effects of gas-stove and microwave-oven emissions to the dangers of excessive noise. Several self-help features are provided to help you improve ventilation, reduce noise, and generally make your environment a more harmonious one. *THE HEALTHY ENVIRONMENT* points out the power that each of us has to improve the quality of our own environment.

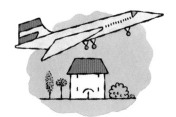

CONTENTS

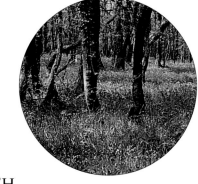

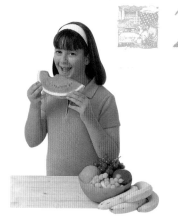

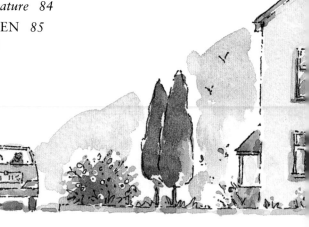

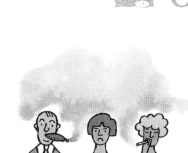

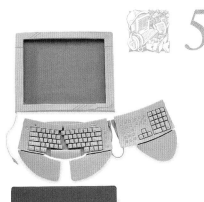

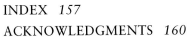

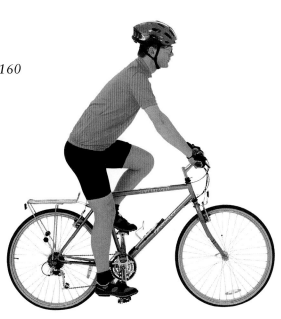

HOW SAFE IS THE WORLD AROUND US?

At times it seems that we are under an ever greater threat from conditions in our environment. How serious are the risks and what can we do about them?

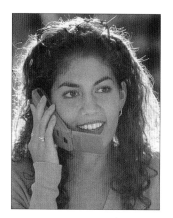

MODERN MENACE?
Although convenient, mobile phones have become a source of irritation in public places, especially in theaters and on public transportation. Users may be irritating more than their neighbors, however; recent research suggests a link between brain tumors and mobile phone use.

OCCUPATIONAL INJURY
Recognized as the father of modern medicine, Hippocrates was the first person known to document occupational hazards.

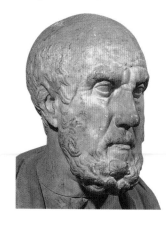

The extent to which our environment is healthy and safe is a subject of major concern to most of us. It seems that almost everywhere we go—our homes, workplaces, social venues, even open outdoor spaces—there is some kind of health threat. People are concerned about the presence of toxic chemicals in drinking water, pesticide residues in food, and the electromagnetic fields produced by electrical transmitters and technological equipment. Even items intended to make our lives easier are under suspicion: cellular phones have recently been linked to serious health issues, including increased incidence of brain tumors, and radiation leaks from microwave ovens have been blamed for causing lymphatic cancer. In the face of so many claims and inconclusive evidence, it can be difficult to establish not only what is hazardous to health but also what realistic steps we can take to minimize any risks. Scientific research projects are underway around the world to assess the actual health risks in a huge number of areas, and governments as well as individuals are paying more attention to the results of such research than ever before.

HEALTH AND SAFETY PIONEERS

We often think of environmental awareness as a relatively recent phenomenon, but in fact, philosophers and scientists alike have long recognized that certain environments can make you unwell. The Greek physician Hippocrates suggested in the fourth century B.C. that illness could result from air contaminated by decaying dead plants and animals, as well as other wastes. He was the first to document an occupational health hazard, reporting that lung diseases were common among the metal diggers of Greece. Today we still use a Greek word, *pneumoconiosis*, to describe a disease caused by the inhalation of dust in an occupational setting. The word literally means "dust in the lungs."

There were also some early attempts to establish environmental regulations. In 13th-century England, laws were passed to eliminate the burning of soft coal, which burns with a smoky yellow flame, because it had been linked to chest complaints. The laws were strict but the practice still continued, even though one unfortunate merchant was hanged in 1306 for burning and selling soft coal.

Many environmental hazards have been ignored by governments and industries, and it has been left to individuals to fight for regulation. Britisher Nellie Kershaw was a victim of the devastating effects of asbestos. She died in 1924 at age 33, having worked for 19 years in an asbestos factory. Despite her doctor's diagnosis of asbestos poisoning as the cause of her ailment, which forced her to give up work, she was denied compensation and benefits by the Friendly Society, to which she had been paying premiums, and also by the government, which claimed that under the Workers' Compensation Act, asbestos poisoning was not listed as an occupational disease. Her

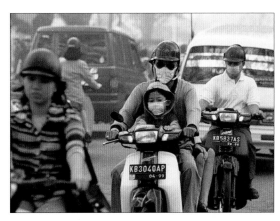

SMOG ALERT
Motorcyclists in Pontianak, Indonesia, wore masks to protect themselves against the smog that covered the region in 1997. One of the worst airborne pollution disasters in history, the smog was caused by fires set to clear forests in the region. Raging uncontrollably for weeks, these fires were doused finally by the monsoon rains.

employer disclaimed liability. Three years after her death she became the first reported case of pulmonary asbestosis, but despite the conclusive evidence, no action was taken to protect other workers. It took until the 1970s for regulatory changes to be enforced in the United Kingdom. Regulations are in effect in other countries, including the United States, but deaths from asbestos persist.

BRINGING ABOUT CHANGE

It has often taken a major disaster to bring about change in response to an environmental health hazard. In October 1948 in Donora, Pennsylvania, 6,000 people became ill and 20 died when a toxic fog enveloped the city for six days. Scientists explained that the unusual weather conditions had combined with Donora's basin topography to trap the pollutants, concentrating them in a harmful cocktail. In London in December 1952, similar foggy conditions trapped pollutants from heavy industry and domestic coal fires to create a lethal pea-soup smog that lasted for five days. The noxious fumes exacerbated conditions such as pneumonia and bronchitis,

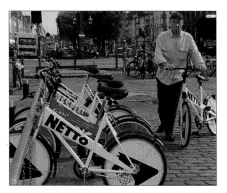

CYCLING SCHEMES
A number of cities in Europe and the United States have introduced bicycle-borrowing schemes that have the dual aim of reducing inner-city vehicle congestion and improving air quality.

SECOND CHANCE
Recycling is one of the most obvious ways that each of us can benefit the planet. Glass containers, metal cans and foil, and all kinds of paper, including newspapers, junk mail, and magazines, are all being recycled in many areas.

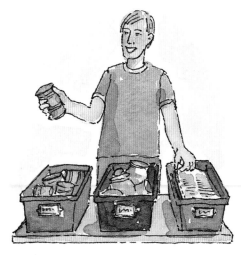

and some 4,000 people died over that period, most of them elderly. Incidents such as these have forced governments to introduce clean air legislation to curb pollution emissions from industry and to ban domestic wood fires and barbecues in some areas. However, we still have a huge amount to learn about improving air quality and reducing pollution. In 1997 smoke from deliberately lit forest fires in Indonesia combined with unusual weather conditions, resulting in a smoke haze that blanketed much of the region for weeks and caused countless respiratory ailments and eye irritations.

Much of the responsibility for the quality of our air rests with all of us; by far the greatest contributor to air pollution is the automobile. Cutting back on its use is the single most important step each of us can take to improve the quality of our environment.

HOPE FOR THE FUTURE

Although the outlook for the environment sometimes appears to be grim, in fact there has been much improvement. Occupational health and safety have become major concerns in most countries, with statutory regulations in place that require workplaces to observe basic guidelines. Recently creative initiatives have been introduced and developed by many countries with the aim of cutting the use of automobiles and encouraging other modes of transportation. For example, some cities—Seattle is one—have made bicycles freely available in city centers. They are electronically tagged to reduce theft and can be borrowed and returned at various sites around the city. Amsterdam and Copenhagen have shown how viable cycling can be as an efficient, healthy mode of transportation. To ensure the safety of cyclists, bicycle lanes are separated from road traffic by a curb, and cyclists have their own traffic lights.

Other initiatives for improving the environment include sophisticated household recycling schemes, studies into nonpolluting forms of energy, and research into effective forms of organic farming that reduce the need for fertilizers, pesticides, and herbicides.

There is also plenty of evidence to show how much can be achieved if the stakes are considered to be sufficiently high. Many people believed that the 1984 Olympics held in Los Angeles would be a disaster because of the dangerously high levels of air pollution common in the city. However, authorities kept vehicles off the roads during critical periods of the competition, which resulted in the ozone levels being dramatically reduced.

A DIFFERENT WAY OF LOOKING AT THE ENVIRONMENT

What environmental scientists have learned in recent years is the extent to which every aspect of the environment is intrinsically interconnected. For instance, no one foresaw that the use of DDT to control malaria-transmitting mosquitoes would have such widespread implications for entire ecosystems and that the chemical could in fact build up to dangerously high levels in animals that it was never intended to affect. Scientists believe that because the chemical compound still persists in the food chain despite having been banned, some humans may have traces of the lethal pesticide in their bodies. Similarly, experts do not attribute the toxic fog of Donora to excess emissions of any one chemical; rather, it was an unpredictable interaction of weather, pollution, and topography that produced the dangerous concoction.

The message seems clear: we need to see ourselves as part of a complex ecosystem and remember that we are as dependent on the general health of that ecosystem as any other creature. Learning to be more in tune with the principles and mechanics of the planet's ecosystems may help us to enjoy an improved lifestyle.

This idea of interconnectedness is the basis of many Eastern philosophies, which state that we are all subject to the influence of universal energy—embodied in everything on the earth—which influences our individual emotions and well-being. This is one of the fundamental principles behind feng shui, the Chinese art of arranging our surroundings to promote well-being.

THE FENG SHUI OF FLOWERS
Feng shui principles can be applied to every aspect of surroundings. Particular flowers placed at certain compass points in your home or workplace are believed to enhance different forms of energy. For example, lilies placed in the northeast corner have a settling influence that can calm an overactive part of the home.

ECO-FRIENDLY GARDENING
Growing your own food, such as tomatoes, herbs, beans, and lettuce, is easy even in the smallest garden. Homegrown produce is tastier and less expensive than supermarket food, and it can be healthier for both you and the environment if you use organic methods.

HEALTHIER WAYS OF LIVING

Although it is easy to feel overwhelmed about the extent of the environmental hazards that we face today, there is in fact a great deal we can do to minimize the potential risks. Many of the common hazards found in the home are well within the control of most people, such as providing adequate ventilation for gas ranges and minimizing allergens. Simple precautions with your food can also reduce the effects of any chemical residues or prevent food poisoning. Thoroughly washing all fruits and vegetables or peeling them, for example, can help to remove most harmful residues.

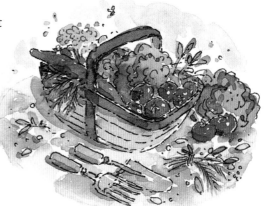

You can make your workplace environment healthier as well. Placing plants that absorb pollution and radiation near photocopiers and computers, for example, will improve air quality. And as a consumer you can make a difference in the quality of your air and water by choosing environmentally friendly cleaning agents. Ultimately, the health of your immediate environment is in your own hands.

WAYS TO A HEALTHY ENVIRONMENT

The aim of this book is to provide straightforward information and practical advice on how to ensure that your environment is healthy.

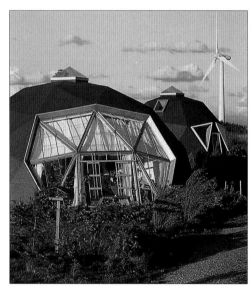

ECO-FRIENDLY HOMES
These domed ecological houses in Denmark make use of many energy-saving and alternative energy-producing devices, such as solar power, water recycling, and wind generators.

It discusses potential hazards that surround us every day, based on the information currently available, and suggests ways of preventing or minimizing risks to your overall health and that of the environment.

Chapter 1 offers a general introduction to a wide range of issues, including how human actions can harm the environment by causing acid rain and global warming. It also shows how small individual actions, such as recycling, can benefit the wider environment.

Chapter 2 concentrates more specifically on each individual element of the environment, including the air we breathe and the water and food we consume. It discusses the potential problems associated with each element and practical solutions for minimizing damage to both ourselves and our environment.

Chapter 3 discusses issues to consider when choosing where to live and the advantages and disadvantages of country, suburban, and urban living. It includes ideas for creating ecologically friendly homes, including the use of solar power and natural building products.

Chapter 4 focuses on the home environment and how to ensure that we minimize potential risks to health through accident or a buildup of pollution. The chapter also shows how to apply the art of feng shui to the layout and interior design of your home.

Most of us have to work, but we don't have to sacrifice our health to our careers. Chapter 5 looks at various working environments and how to avoid common occupational health problems.

Finally, Chapter 6 covers issues that surround popular places of leisure. It gives helpful tips on safety while traveling at home and abroad and provides advice on how to avoid risks both to your own health and to the environment while still living life to the fullest.

How can you ensure that your environment is healthy?

The various hazards that the environment poses to health are constantly examined in the media. Everything seems to be bad for us; the food we eat, the water we drink and the air we breathe, all seem to be the subjects of frequent health scares. There are many things that we, as individuals, can do to protect our own health and well-being, and to make sure that the wider environment is as safe and pleasant as possible.

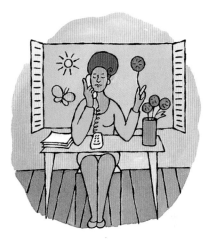

Q **ARE YOU GENERALLY HEALTHY BUT SUFFER FROM UNEXPLAINED SYMPTOMS AT WORK?**
You could be afflicted by sick building syndrome (see Chapter 5). Common symptoms include lethargy, headaches, itchy eyes, and poor ability to concentrate. The syndrome, though it is not a recognized illness, can have a number of causes—from toxins within the workplace to workers' attitudes toward their jobs. Certain steps can be taken to relieve the symptoms, such as improving ventilation to expel any stale air and introducing plants to absorb the toxins from electrical equipment.

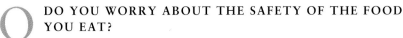

Q **DO YOU WORRY ABOUT THE SAFETY OF THE FOOD YOU EAT?**
Recent reports about outbreaks of *E. coli* and salmonella poisoning have alerted people to the whole issue of food safety. Chapter 2 suggests methods of buying and storing foods so that the chances of developing food poisoning are minimized, and also discusses the health risks posed by the pesticides and fertilizers used in modern farming, as well as any health implications of additives and food contaminants.

Q **ARE YOU PLANNING TO MOVE BUT CAN'T DECIDE ON THE TYPE OF LOCATION?**
There are many factors to consider when moving (see Chapter 3). It is commonly believed that country living is better for general health and well-being than urban living because of the fresh air and slower pace of life. However, pollution in the country, whether from agricultural pesticides or natural radon radiation, can be just as harmful as in urban areas. Furthermore, the loneliness often experienced in quiet rural retreats can cause a great deal of stress in some people. All these factors and more need to be taken into account when deciding where to live.

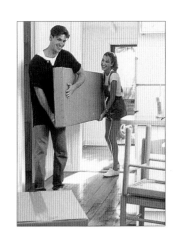

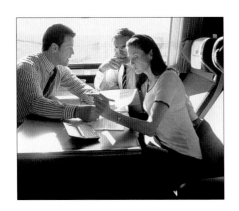

Q DOES THE AMOUNT OF POLLUTION IN THE AIR CAUSE YOU CONCERN?

Scientists are investigating the extent to which a worldwide increase in the incidence of asthma may be linked to air quality. Most people accept, however, that a reduction in vehicle emissions is in everyone's interest. Alternative modes of transportation, such as buses and trains, can greatly reduce the amount of toxic car fumes in the air, while cycling and walking have the added benefit of improving people's fitness levels. Air quality issues are examined in Chapter 2.

Q ARE YOU INTERESTED IN FENG SHUI BUT NOT SURE HOW TO APPLY IT IN YOUR OWN HOME?

Feng shui is the Chinese art of designing and arranging a home to promote health, wealth, and happiness. It is a practical system based partly on common sense and partly on the principle that an underlying cosmological energy force inhabits and rules over everything. The aim of feng shui is to optimize the flow of this energy, or chi, throughout your home. Chapter 4 provides some practical guidelines on how to arrange individual rooms in your home in order to encourage good health, well-being, and success.

Q ARE YOU WORRIED THAT YOUR HOME MAY HAVE ACCIDENTS WAITING TO HAPPEN?

Accidents within the home are the most common cause of injury, especially among young children. Most of these injuries can be prevented by being aware of potential hazards and taking simple precautions (see Chapter 4). Children are naturally inquisitive, so locking away harmful substances and keeping children away from danger zones, such as stairways, is essential. There are also many gadgets available to help maintain safety in the home.

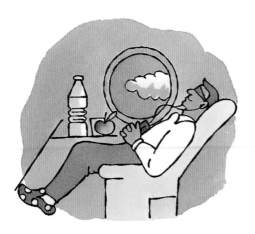

Q DO YOU ENJOY TRAVELING BUT WORRY ABOUT THE HEALTH RISKS INVOLVED?

Travel abroad is an enriching experience, but it can pose health risks. Travel-related diseases, such as malaria, are on the increase, and the risk of poisoning from contaminated food and water is widespread in many regions. Air travel also causes problems; jet lag can result in fatigue, insomnia, anxiety and diminished ability to concentrate, which can often lead to stress or an accident. Chapter 6 offers some practical advice on how to minimize health risks while traveling.

CHAPTER 1

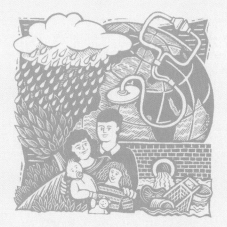

YOUR ENVIRONMENT

*A healthy environment is fundamental
to a good standard of living. We can all
contribute to improving our surroundings,
first by being aware of the many environmental
problems that the world faces today and second
by supporting green initiatives, such as recycling
schemes. By adapting our lifestyles, often in
simple ways, we can improve both our own
health and that of the environment.*

HOW HEALTHY IS YOUR ENVIRONMENT?

Your environment is integral to your quality of life. Taking steps to improve your living conditions by enhancing the good aspects and reducing the harmful ones can benefit your health.

The environment affects health and well-being in three ways—physically, mentally, and spiritually. Perhaps because the impact of a healthy environment on physical and mental health is easier to detect, its importance for spiritual well-being is often overlooked in Western societies. But according to many Eastern views, including traditional Chinese medicine and the Indian medical practice of Ayurveda, good health can be achieved only if you are in harmony with the environment. Being out of step with the world around you can lead to internal imbalances and upset your spiritual well-being, which in turn may lead to physical and mental disorders.

Increasingly, however, people in the Western world are coming to accept that each individual is an integral part of a wider environment. There is a growing conviction that unhealthy home and workplace conditions; polluted streams, rivers, lakes, and oceans; destroyed woodlands; and poor air quality can diminish your quality of life on a spiritual level, as well as damage your mental and physical health.

UNIVERSAL ENERGY

In the East, many cultures share a belief in an eternal life force flowing throughout the entire universe, affecting and interacting with all aspects of our environment. In China this energy is called chi (the written symbol is shown below); in Japan it is known as ki. Achieving balance and harmony with this life force, seen as a movement of electromagnetic energy, is the basis of Oriental philosophy and medicine.

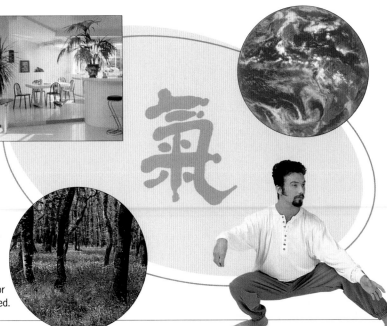

Buildings have their own flow of chi. Those made of synthetic materials and sealed to the elements can be physically draining and mentally disorienting, while those constructed from natural materials can be invigorating.

Each season has a different flow of energy. Spring and summer have dynamic, expansive yang energy, while autumn and winter have passive, inward-turning yin energy. The Chinese identify a fifth season at the end of summer that is neither yin nor yang but is perfectly balanced.

The planet has chi that extends outside its physical mass and is known as the earth's force. It flows constantly, carried by wind, water, light, and sound. Chi also flows to the earth from other planets and the galaxy, which is known as heaven's force.

The body has chi that flows through it like blood and extends up to three feet beyond the body as an aura. This personal chi mixes with environmental chi. To retain your own vital energy, it is important that your environment be as healthy as possible.

THE RISE IN FOOD POISONING

Each year between 24 and 81 million cases of food poisoning occur in the United States. The numbers have been steadily rising, but food safety experts say the true figures are hard to determine because so many cases go unreported or are mistaken for other ailments. Seven of the most common causes of food-borne illness are the bacteria salmonella, *E. coli, C. jejuni, C. perfringens, S. aureus, B. cereus,* and listeria. The first four bacteria are most often ingested in meat and poultry dishes, but salmonella also occurs in fish and eggs. *S. aureus* produces a heat-stable toxin in meat and seafood salads, sandwich spreads, and high-salt foods that have been improperly stored. *B. cereus* grows in starchy foods, such as pasta, rice, and potato dishes. Listeria thrives in milk, soft cheeses, and vegetables fertilized with manure.

As an individual there are three principal ways you can improve your environment: behave in an ecologically responsible way, set an example for others, and put pressure on your local and national governments to adopt pro-environment policies. A first step is to be clear about what exactly is meant by the word *environment*. One dictionary defines it as "the circumstances, objects, or conditions by which one is surrounded." This term applies equally to your own home, workplace, town, and its surrounding countryside, as well as the rest of the world.

IN THE HOME AND WORKPLACE

It is often possible to find solutions to environmental problems, once you recognize the link between them and health. For example, fumes from gas stoves, furnaces, and space and water heaters can provoke chronic breathing disorders, and many deaths are caused each year by carbon monoxide from gas appliances. Keeping your home well ventilated and your appliances properly maintained can prevent such occurrences.

Persistent dampness is another problem. The minute droppings of dust mites, tiny creatures that thrive in warm, damp conditions, can irritate the breathing passages in sensitive people and trigger asthma attacks.

In the kitchen, poor hygiene, inefficient storage methods, and undercooking of meat and poultry greatly increase the risk of food poisoning. Statistics show this risk to be rising. It is believed to result partly from factory farming methods, which help promote the spread of harmful organisms, and partly from the increased popularity of fast foods, which may not have been cooked sufficiently to kill harmful bacteria or may have been held at temperatures that encourage their growth.

The most common symptom of food poisoning is diarrhea, often accompanied by abdominal cramps and nausea. Symptoms usually arise within 12 to 24 hours of eating contaminated food and subside within a day or two. In the majority of people food poisoning is a minor incident, but for infants, the elderly, and anyone with a compromised immune system, it can be very serious.

Measures you can take to prevent food poisoning include washing your hands and food preparation surfaces and utensils before and after handling raw foods and keeping refrigerated foods below 40°F and hot foods above 140°F. Holding foods at room temperature, except for those that are highly acidified with lemon juice or vinegar, is a sure way to promote bacterial growth.

Another environmental problem in the home and workplace is radon, a naturally occurring radioactive gas released from rocks, water, and soil. Regular exposure to radon has health effects similar to smoking 10 cigarettes a day. In fact, radon is now established as the most common cause of lung cancer among nonsmokers. This gas is found everywhere but is a particular problem in areas where it exists naturally in high concentrations. The main danger occurs when there is a buildup of radon inside a building, but measures can be taken to reduce or eliminate the risk (see page 57).

Excessive noise disturbance is another growing concern in many urban areas. Although laws exist to protect people from the disruptive behavior of others, many people are reluctant to inform on their neighbors. Some local authorities have set up noise patrols to combat the problem and prosecute persistent offenders.

Noise from road traffic and maintenance, aircraft, and industry can also have a damaging effect on health. Research indicates that people living near airports and busy highways may suffer two to three times the

Noise nuisance
Pollution is not limited just to toxic substances. Noise can be unhealthy, as well as disturbing.

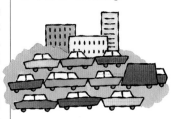

ROAD TRAFFIC NOISE
Constant traffic noise can cause anxiety and stress-related illness.

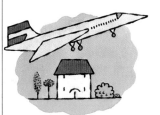

AIRCRAFT NOISE
Living under a flight path can affect your health and well-being.

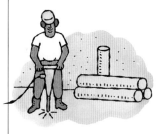

INDUSTRIAL NOISE
Precautions against excessive noise are essential in certain jobs.

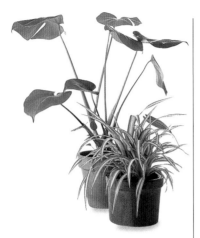

HELPFUL PLANTS
Plants can be an easy and inexpensive way to make a working environment healthier. They keep the air more humid, and a few actually mop up certain pollutants.

average level of anxiety and stress-related conditions such as high blood pressure, not to mention constant sleep disturbance, as those who live in quieter areas. (See pages 62–65 for more information on noise.)

The working environment

In the workplace the threat to health may come from toxic chemicals and gases, as well as harmful substances such as asbestos and textiles. These can cause lung disorders, including asbestosis, pneumoconiosis, and emphysema. Caustic chemicals can bring on skin and breathing disorders, and constant excessive noise levels can lead to temporary hearing loss, even permanent deafness.

Office workers can suffer from a condition referred to as "sick building syndrome." This is a collection of ill-health effects believed to be related to poor building design and construction, inadequate ventilation, badly maintained air conditioning, and chemical emissions from furnishings and technological equipment (see pages 121–123).

All working environments are covered by health and safety laws, but this legislation is effective only when individuals follow safe working practices and report serious breaches of the rules to management, a workers' representative, an environmental health officer (see page 24), or the state or local agency that is responsible for overseeing the particular violation.

Public buildings and recreational venues

Public buildings pose other environmental hazards. There are laws covering many aspects of health and safety in public venues, and individuals have an important part to play in reporting problems to public health organizations.

In hospitals there is always concern about the spread of infection. Because the immune system of patients, in particular sick children, the elderly, and those recovering from major surgery, is lowered, they have a reduced ability to combat disease, making infection especially dangerous. One of the most serious problems is a strain of *Staphylococcus* bacteria that has become resistant to a wide range of antibiotics.

In restaurants and bars customers are often forced to breathe in other people's tobacco smoke—known as passive smoking (see page 136)—which increases their risk

HOW BACTERIA BECOME RESISTANT TO DRUGS

Increased use of antibiotics, both in human medicine and animal farming practice, may be contributing to a new league of illnesses that are resistant to antibiotics as treatment. This is because bacteria grow and multiply incredibly quickly—a single bacterium can become a colony of 250,000 in just six hours.

Over several generations bacteria can adapt their growth and reproductive cycles by natural selection to resist an antibiotic or develop an enzyme that blocks its action. These drug-resistant strains of bacteria can be very problematic in hospitals, where they pose a special risk to immune-deficient patients.

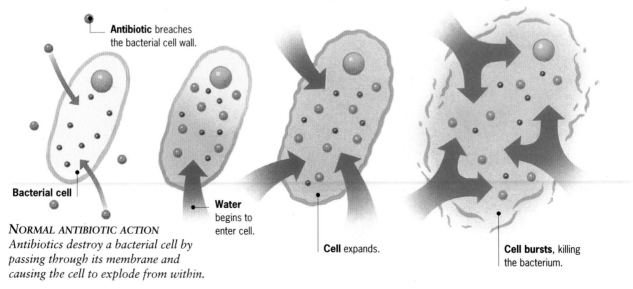

Antibiotic breaches the bacterial cell wall.

Bacterial cell

NORMAL ANTIBIOTIC ACTION
Antibiotics destroy a bacterial cell by passing through its membrane and causing the cell to explode from within.

Water begins to enter cell.

Cell expands.

Cell bursts, killing the bacterium.

of lung cancer, heart disease, and respiratory problems. Many restaurants and bars now have segregated smoking areas, and an increasing number of local and state ordinances prohibit smoking in bars and many public buildings.

Nightclubs, discos, and bars pose additional environmental risks, including excessively high noise levels from sound systems, which can cause both temporary hearing loss and permanent damage to ears.

Water quality

Unsafe drinking water is one of the leading global health problems. At least 900 million cases of diarrhea occur every year from the drinking of contaminated water, and more than 4 million children die annually from waterborne diseases. But the effect that water quality has on our physical health and well-being is sometimes difficult to quantify. In 1988 aluminum sulfate was accidentally added to the water supply at Camelford, in Cornwall, England, and was followed by widespread reports of disorders such as digestive and kidney problems. Creeks, rivers, and lakes can also be contaminated by toxic substances seeping into ground water from septic tanks.

Excess fertilizer and slurry from farmland and sewage from badly located runoffs can encourage the excess growth of algae. These so-called algal blooms produce powerful toxins that can harm wildlife, domestic pets, and humans who bathe in the water. Such contamination can also lead to oxygen reduction in the waterways, resulting in the suffocation of fish.

The Environmental Protection Agency (EPA) and state and local governments have set high standards to ensure that water is suitable for human consumption. However, there is increasing concern among many individuals about the minuscule amounts of toxic chemicals that may still enter the domestic water supply and have an adverse effect on people's health. They include lead, pesticides, nitrates, dioxins (waste products from certain manufacturing processes and waste incineration), arsenic, and alkyl phenols, which are found in some detergents. There is also concern about some of the chemicals used to treat water—chlorine, for example—which can convert to toxic substances. (See pages 42–45 for more information on water quality.)

FEEDING THE WEEDS

One common cause of water pollution is excessive plant nutrients, which feed algae and other water plants, so that they grow out of control. These nutrients—essentially nitrogen, phosphorus, and potassium— occur naturally in limited amounts, and so plant growth is limited. But excess levels in the runoff from fertilized agricultural land, industrial waste (particularly chemical effluents), and human sewage have led to rivers and lakes being choked by algal blooms and the fish eventually dying through suffocation.

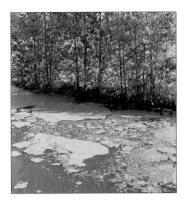

ALGAL BLOOMS
This freshwater stream in Britain has been polluted by fertilizers and industrial waste. The algal blooms proliferate at the expense of other water plants and fish.

THE WIDER ENVIRONMENT

Within the wider environment, perhaps the most important factor that can make a difference to your health is where you live (see page 75). It makes sense, if you can, to choose a location away from congested roads and heavy industry or other areas where atmospheric and landscape conditions encourage a buildup of polluted air.

Traffic fumes, which can cause or aggravate respiratory problems, such as asthma and bronchitis, are being increasingly linked also with cardiorespiratory (heart and lung) disorders. Carbon monoxide (CO), one of the by-products of car exhaust, is thought to be one of the pollutants responsible for heart disorders, mainly because it reduces the blood's ability to transport oxygen

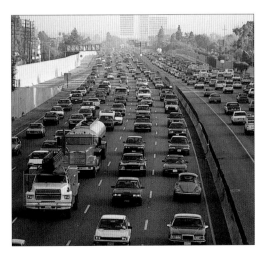

TRAFFIC POLLUTION
Traffic fumes today are one of the major causes of air pollution. During the summer especially, pollution levels can build up to dangerously high levels. The action of sunlight causes a reaction between nitrogen dioxide in the air and the hydrocarbons from the exhausts of motor vehicles, resulting in ground-level ozone pollution.

TRAFFIC AND AIR POLLUTION

Automobile traffic is the main source of air pollution today, contributing both primary pollutants (toxic gases released directly into the air) and secondary pollutants (formed when primary pollutants interact with other gases in the atmosphere). Some are by-products from the incomplete combustion of fuel in the sealed environment of an engine. In traffic jams the occupants of motor vehicles are exposed to twice as much pollution as pedestrians or cyclists on the same road, mostly because the car draws in air from the exhaust pipe of the car in front. Keeping a window partially open helps to keep air circulating.

AIR POLLUTION Traffic fumes contain harmful chemicals that are the main cause of air pollution today.

1, Carbon monoxide prevents blood from carrying oxygen throughout the body.

1, Benzene is carcinogenic.

1, Hydrocarbons include some carcinogenic substances.

1, Sulfur dioxide can lead to breathing problems.

1, Carbon dioxide is a greenhouse gas. Large levels of it in the atmosphere contribute to global warming.

2, Low-level ozone irritates the eyes, nose, throat, and airways, causing coughing, headache, and chest pain. It can aggravate lung problems, such as asthma.

1, Lead harms the nervous system and retards mental development. It is especially harmful to children.

1, Particulates are carcinogenic and may aggravate breathing conditions such as asthma.

1 or 2, Nitrogen dioxide affects the airways. It can cause breathing problems and aggravate lung conditions, such as emphysema and asthma.

1=primary pollutant   **2**=secondary pollutant

around the body. Ground-level ozone (CO_3), caused by the action of sunlight on car exhaust, is also strongly linked to respiratory disorders and heart disease. And recent studies in the United States suggest that particulates, small particles of soot and other bits of solid materials released into the air by poorly maintained diesel engines, may be responsible for the deaths of 2,000 city dwellers every year.

But automobiles are not the only culprits when it comes to noxious emissions that cause respiratory problems; the small hand-held engines in lawn and garden equipment, such as trimmers and chainsaws, contribute about one-tenth of the hydrocarbon pollution in the United States. New standards for this equipment became effective in 1997, and by 2007 improvements in emission controls are expected to cut pollution caused by handheld garden engines by 70 percent.

One of the most important ways that we can all help to improve the general level of our air quality is to keep our own car use to a minimum. There are many alternatives, such as forming a car pool, using public transportation, and walking or bicycling whenever possible. The last two can be of benefit not only to the environment but also to your general fitness level. You can also encourage local authorities to switch to low-polluting forms of public transportation, such as electric buses (see page 71).

Significant steps have been taken to improve general air quality in the United States since 1955, when the first Air Pollution Control Act was passed by Congress; it has been amended several times since, most recently in 1990. While the law sets minimum standards for air quality throughout the nation, states and metropolitan areas can set more stringent standards if they choose, and many of them have. But there is still much work to be done.

There is compelling evidence that carbon dioxide and other so-called greenhouse gases (GHG) are causing climate changes at an alarming rate. At a meeting in Kyoto, Japan, in 1997, legally binding limits on GHG emissions were set for 38 industrialized countries, to begin between 2008 and 2012. The United States has agreed to reduce its carbon emissions by 7 percent below its 1990 emission levels in that period. Many energy-efficient measures must be put in place to meet this target.

ENVIRONMENTAL HEALTH

We can all play a part in promoting environmental health by recognizing the need for proper hygiene and making sure that our actions do not create pollution.

Many aspects of environmental health that we take for granted today, such as clean water and efficient waste disposal, date only from the late 1800s and result from the efforts of a few concerned individuals. Throughout most of the 19th century, living conditions for the working classes were appalling in most Western countries. Overcrowding in particular was a major problem. A Liverpool housing survey in 1846 found that 30,000 people lived in dank, dingy cellars without running water.

There were few controls on working conditions either, especially in factories. Men, women, and children were required to toil for long hours in hot, damp, and badly ventilated manufacturing facilities and mines. There was no proper sanitation, and machinery was dangerous and unguarded.

Much of the working population was badly malnourished, and there was no attempt to regulate food standards. Certain foodstuffs, such as bread, were routinely adulterated with alum and other substances, and milk, beer, and spirits were diluted with water—often from polluted wells.

Many wells and rivers were contaminated with sewage from houses and factories. Consequently, the population suffered epidemics of waterborne diseases, such as typhoid and cholera; a cholera outbreak in 1832 claimed 22,000 lives in London alone. Overcrowding in urban areas throughout North America and Europe meant that contagious diseases like scarlet fever, tuberculosis, and diphtheria were rife. Mortality rates were highest among children—30 percent of infants died before age five. These repeated epidemics led to international sanitary conventions, held in Europe between 1851 and 1892. The conventions evolved into the Health Organization of the League of Nations in 1919, which in 1948 became the World Health Organization (WHO), an agency of the United Nations.

Green initiative

The ZEUS program, a Europe-wide scheme aimed at introducing alternatively fueled vehicles to city centers, was first implemented in 1996. Its aim was to buy and operate more than 1,000 zero- and low-emission fleet vehicles—from electrically powered cars and buses to bicycles— within three years.

DID YOU KNOW?

In the 1900s the practice of adulterating food with foreign substances was so common that many people forgot the taste of natural food. Cooperative societies that were committed to providing pure food and fair service believed that the public disliked the look and taste of unadulterated produce. One society even educated its members about the real flavor of tea.

LEGIONNAIRES' DISEASE

Legionnaires' disease is named after an outbreak of a severe illness in 1976 that caused the deaths of 29 members of the American Legion attending a convention in Philadelphia. The infection, which causes pneumonia-like symptoms, is thought to be caught by inhaling contaminated droplets from air-conditioning systems or showers. Water systems in public buildings are now rigorously disinfected, but there are still many cases of the disease every year. The elderly and heavy smokers are most at risk.

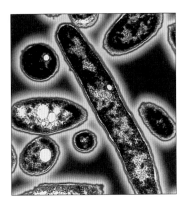

LEGIONELLA PNEUMOPHILA
The bacterium that causes Legionnaires' disease is a common contaminant of water systems in public buildings.

Environmental reforms

The Industrial Revolution of the 18th century in the United Kingdom led to the introduction of new living standards laws. These were adopted by many developed countries all over the world. Most of the improvements introduced were due to the efforts of the social reformer Sir Edwin Chadwick. His investigations led to the 1833 Factory Act, which mandated compulsory schooling and a reduction in the working hours of children, as well as the provision of adequate sanitation. The act set up salaried factory inspectors who ensured that dangerous machinery was fenced off and that conditions reached minimum standards of health and hygiene.

Chadwick's main achievement, however, was in public health. He was largely responsible for the 1848 Public Health Act in

Creative recycling

Old newspapers and magazines can be recycled creatively by making papier-mâché with them. Here is the basic technique for making a bowl.

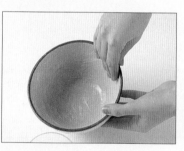

1 To prepare the mold, choose a bowl and coat it with petroleum jelly to prevent the papier-mâché from sticking.

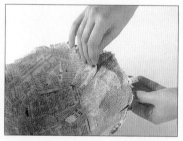

2 Tear newspaper into small strips, dip them in wallpaper paste, and apply about eight layers of these to the inside of the mold.

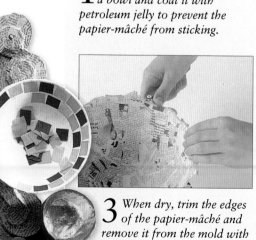

3 When dry, trim the edges of the papier-mâché and remove it from the mold with a knife.

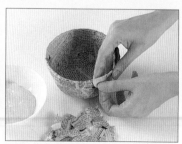

4 Neaten the edges of the bowl by covering it with strips of paper. When dry, coat it with poster paint and lacquer if desired.

LITTER

Litter is a serious problem worldwide in both urban and rural areas, and its effects can be very far-reaching. For example, turtles in the Pacific Ocean have been suffocated by floating plastic bags, which look similar to the jellyfish on which they feed.

Even though littering is a punishable offense nationwide, much work still needs to be done to stem the rising tide of refuse along city streets and highways, on waterways and beaches, and in public parks. You can do your part by not littering and by signing up every year for the spring cleanup in your community or organizing one if none is yet underway.

Britain, which made drains and sanitation a requirement in all new homes. Henceforth, public streets had to be paved, drained, and cleaned; slaughter plants and rooming houses had to be registered; and basements under 6½ feet high were banned as residences.

ENVIRONMENTAL HEALTH TODAY

In most Western countries a range of legislation covers all aspects of environmental health. Particular concern is paid to food safety; the production, manufacture, and sale of foods is usually tightly controlled. In the United States stringent regulations govern food production—from farming practices to hygiene in restaurants. Their adequate enforcement depends on the employment of sufficient numbers of well-trained inspectors to carry out regular inspections. The agencies responsible for environmental health include the Environmental Protection Agency (EPA) and local health departments.

Food monitoring

Several tests are used to monitor levels of food contamination. Foods are checked for industrial chemicals, heavy metals, radioactivity, nitrates and nitrites; farming residues, such as pesticides and hormones; the effects of manufacturing practices, such as adding coloring and preservatives; contamination from bacteria and packaging materials; and the level of naturally occurring toxins, such as aflatoxin, a black mold found on peanuts.

continued on page 26

A QUICK GUIDE TO CONTROVERSIAL FOOD ADDITIVES

Many people believe that almost all food additives are bad and should be avoided, but a number are natural substances that have been used for hundreds of years with no ill effects. Many additives, in fact, enhance food safety by inhibiting the growth of food-poisoning bacteria and preventing spoilage from oxidation of fats.

The Center for Food Safety and Applied Nutrition, an arm of the U.S. Food and Drug Administration, is responsible for approving and regulating the thousands of additives used in food manufacturing, cosmetics, and drugs. Although the ones they approve have been tested extensively and proven to be safe, some do cause unpleasant symptoms in people who are sensitive to them. If you suffer from allergies, you could have reactions to additives. A few other additives are controversial because experiments have shown them to be possible causes of other health problems, such as eye damage or cancer, when ingested in large amounts. Several additives, their common uses, and their possible effects are listed below.

COMMON NAME	COMMON USES	MAY CAUSE
Colorings		
FD&C Yellow #5 (tartrazine)	Cereals, puddings, ice cream, soft drinks, breakfast cereals, candy, bakery products, some drugs, hair rinses, bath salts	Can cause allergic reactions, including hives and asthma.
Cochineal (carmine)	Fruit drinks, frozen pops, candy, cosmetics	May provoke allergic reactions.
Caramel	Sauces, gravies, soft drinks	When processed with sulfites, may cause reactions in people who are sensitive to sulfites.
Annatto	Potato chips, cereals, snack foods	May provoke asthma and rashes.
Canthaxanthin	Feed for chickens and farmed salmon; tablets to enhance tanning	May cause eye damage when taken as tablets for tanning.
Preservatives		
Benzoic acid	Fruit products, beverages, ice cream	May cause asthma, rashes, red eyes.
Sulfites	Dried fruits and vegetables, wine	May provoke asthma, hives, diarrhea, nausea.
Butylated hydroxyanisole (BHA) Butylated hydroxytoluene (BHT)	Beef stock cubes, cheese spreads, margarine, cake mixes, potato chips	May provoke hives. Have been linked to increased cancer risk and liver enlargement.
Parabens	Processed foods, cosmetics, drugs	May cause dermatitis and anaphylactic shock.
Flavor enhancers		
Disodium 5-guanulate	Canned soups, meat, sauces, spreads	May cause allergic reactions.
Monosodium glutamate	Chinese food, soups, stews, snack foods	May cause burning skin, headache, nausea, heart palpitations, weakness, and dizziness.
Emulsifiers, thickeners		
Carageenan	Milk shakes, ice cream, quick-setting jelly mixtures	Linked to ulcers in the colon. Large amounts have caused fetal damage in test animals.
Gum tragacanth	Salad dressings, pie fillings, ice cream	May cause allergic reactions.
Sweeteners		
Sorbitol, mannitol, xylitol	Sugar-free candy and chewing gum	May have a laxative effect in large amounts.
Acesulfame-K, aspartame, saccharin, sucralose	Soft drinks, yogurt, and other products labeled "sugar free"	Have possible links to cancer and brain and nerve disorders. Some people have reported sensitivity.

The Public Health Professional

Public health professionals have the vital jobs not only of protecting public health but also of safeguarding the quality of the environment and working with local, state, national, and international health organizations on vital health issues.

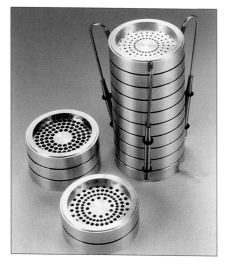

AIR MONITORS
A cascade impactor for particle sizing, shown here, is a monitor that checks pollution levels in the air. Air is pumped through the device, and at each level a certain size of particle is filtered out.

Public health professionals are responsible for ensuring that the health and well-being of the communities in which they serve are of a high standard. Some offer advice on health and safety matters and enforce public health legislation. Others do research on the cause, treatment, control, and prevention of disease. Still others work on programs to promote better mental health care or combat drug and alcohol abuse and other health hazards. And many are involved in programs that monitor air quality, water purity, and sanitary conditions in food and beverage businesses.

Where do public health professionals work?

Public health employees may work for any of the eight agencies of the federal Public Health Service (PHS): the Agency for Health Care Policy and Research, the Agency for Toxic Substances and Disease Registry, the Centers for Disease Control and Prevention, the Food and Drug Administration, the Indian Health Service, the Health Resources and Services Administration, the National Institutes of Health, or the Substance Abuse and Mental Health Services Administration. All of these organizations are under the umbrella of the U.S. Department of Health and Human Services.

Some health professionals are also military or civilian employees of the Public Health Service Commissioned Corps, a branch of the armed services, which assigns officers to the Environmental Protection Agency and other government organizations that deal with public health issues.

Others are employed in industry— with food manufacturers and supermarket chains, for example. Some also work as health and safety inspectors for local health departments. Still others monitor

Origins

A movement to improve public health in Britain arose in response to appalling living conditions in the 19th century. Industrialization and a switch from largely rural to urban living were responsible for chronic overcrowding, poor sanitation and water supplies, and the spread of diseases such as cholera.

In 1842 Sir Edwin Chadwick published a damning report on the sanitary conditions of the laboring population. This led to the 1848 Public Health Act, which established local boards of health to improve water and sewage systems, curb health nuisances, and halt the spread of disease.

In the United States a national health agency grew out of the Marine Hospital Service, which was established in 1798. It was

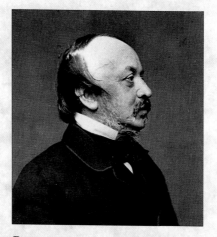

PIONEER IN PUBLIC HEALTH
Sir Edwin Chadwick (1800–1890) launched the public health movement in Great Britain with his report on intolerable living conditions.

renamed the Public Health Service in 1912 and is today part of the Department of Health and Human Services.

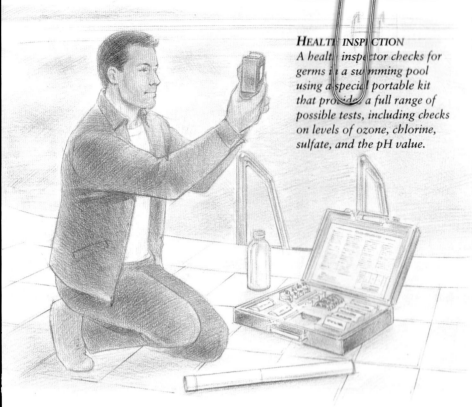

HEALTH INSPECTION
A health inspector checks for germs in a swimming pool using a special portable kit that provides a full range of possible tests, including checks on levels of ozone, chlorine, sulfate, and the pH value.

What other work do public health professionals do?

Some public health professionals investigate outbreaks of infections such as salmonella and Legionnaires' disease and organize emergency control measures as appropriate. Many do research into the causes and treatments of such diseases. Others work for social service agencies that deal with health care issues.

Do public health professionals safeguard the local environment?

There are environmental specialists who monitor the purity of tap water or the condition of water in public swimming pools as part of their duties. Others are involved in overseeing the disposal of hazardous waste, investigating illegal dumping, and perhaps having offenders prosecuted.

What qualifications do public health professionals have?

Most public health professionals have a university degree in either environmental studies or public health. Many have advanced degrees in one of these subjects as well.

working conditions in offices and in leisure and service businesses, investigating incidents involving health and safety; they may advise managers on improving training and work procedures.

Most public health professionals specialize in a particular subject area—for example, health and safety in the workplace or control of pollution and other environmental hazards.

How do health inspectors work?

People who specialize in monitoring public health conditions usually work for local health departments. They can enter a business in order to investigate a possible offense and, when necessary, take away samples for examination. When monitoring food safety, for example, they carry out regular unannounced inspections of food factories, butcher shops, restaurants, cafes, delicatessens, and other eating establishments.

In addition to giving advice on food handling and hygiene, a public health inspector can enforce measures to control infestations of pests such as rats and cockroaches in commercial enterprises and can order

that improvements be carried out in substandard premises. In serious cases they can even close down an offending business until corrections have been made.

WHAT YOU CAN DO AT HOME

Storing food in a refrigerator prolongs its life because cold air slows the growth of bacteria, but the temperature must be kept at the proper level (see below). Dated products can be kept until the sell-by date and up to a week beyond. Keeping times for some other foods are listed below; they vary depending on freshness when purchased.

FOOD TYPE	KEEPS FOR	FOOD TYPE	KEEPS FOR
Fish	24 hours	Eggs, hard cooked	1 week
Meat, ground	1 to 2 days	Lettuce, spinach	3 to 5 days
Poultry	2 to 4 days	Cheese, semihard	2 to 3 months
Peppers, tomatoes	1 week	Jams and spreads	2 months
Apples	2 to 3 weeks	Butter	2 to 4 weeks

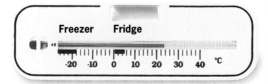

Freezer   Fridge

-20   -10   0   10   20   30   40   °C

REFRIGERATING FOOD
To keep food fresh, a freezer should be set at -18°C (0°F) or lower, and a refrigerator should be kept between 1° and 4°C (34° and 40°F).

Following the Chernobyl nuclear reactor disaster in 1986, food is now checked for radioactivity in many European countries. Radioactive fallout from Chernobyl is still found in samples, but most radioactivity in food comes from natural sources and is at a level currently considered acceptable.

The term *pesticide* covers not only chemicals used to kill or repel insects but also those employed to control rats and mice (rodenticides), weeds (herbicides), fungus and molds (fungicides), algae (algicides), viruses and bacteria (disinfectants), and weeds (herbicides). Also considered pesticides are defoliants, desiccants, insect-growth regulators, and plant-growth regulators.

Pesticides must have undergone extensive testing before approval and must have standards for how they are stored and applied and how much time must be allowed between application and harvesting. In use they must meet strict pesticide residue limits, or tolerances. This is the amount allowed on food to ensure that even if large quantities are eaten, the quantity consumed will have no ill effects. The Food Quality and Protection Act, passed in 1996, requires a reevaluation of all tolerances for residues in both raw and processed foods within 10 years.

All the above stipulations are overseen in this country by the Environmental Protection Agency (EPA), but other government agencies, both federal and local, monitor food to be sure that it meets standards. For example, the Food and Drug Administration (FDA) and the U.S. Department of Agriculture (USDA) check for residues in all food involved in interstate commerce.

AIR, WATER, AND LAND QUALITY

Air, water, and land pollution are rarely confined within political borders, which is why the International Federation of Environmental Health (IFEH) was established. Some health problems span several countries. Within the IFEH four regional groups deal with localized environmental health problems. The regional groups are Africa, North and South America, Euro/Asia/Pacific Rim, and Scandinavia. The IFEH works with the World Health Organization (WHO) to help create a healthy global environment.

Waste gas and smoke emissions from heavy industry are monitored by individual governments and the WHO. The United Nations Commission on Human Settlements, known as Habitat, has also been involved. At a 1999 conference in Nairobi, Kenya, delegates approved a resolution to phase out leaded gasoline. (The United States is among several countries that are already lead free.) Some 20 percent of gasoline worldwide still has to be converted.

Air quality in the United States is monitored by the EPA. Its agents are concerned with the amounts of principal, or criteria, air pollutants that are considered harmful. These include low-level ozone (see page 39), sulfur dioxide, nitrogen oxides, and particulates (dust, soot, and other bits of solid material). States and local authorities usually monitor air quality, and when levels of certain pollutants reach dangerous levels, they issue warnings. For example, when ozone levels are high, public announcements advise people with respiratory disorders to stay indoors and/or seek a doctor's advice. Some environmental groups believe that ozone limits are set too high and recommend that health warnings be issued sooner.

Setting standards for safe drinking water and monitoring public water utilities come under the jurisdiction of the EPA as well. While the agency has already set maximum contaminant levels (MCLs) for about 100 contaminants found in the nation's water supplies, they still have to set standards for hundreds more that have been identified.

The EPA also regulates the treatment and disposal of hazardous waste and the management and restoration of contaminated land sites. The disposal of certain toxic and radioactive wastes, which remain harmful for 300 to several million years, presents special problems that need to be addressed.

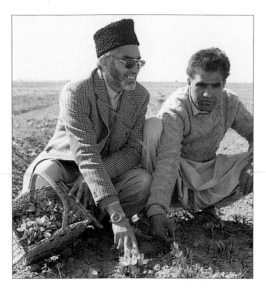

SAFETY AT WORK
Many governments protect their workforce by imposing safety criteria and limiting exposure to harmful substances. Different cultures have different health problems. Saffron pickers, like these Kashmiri men, can suffer harmful effects on mental health from gases emitted by saffron. In Iran the working hours of saffron pickers are restricted.

GLOBAL ISSUES

By understanding the global implications of our actions, we can learn to behave in ways that inflict less damage on the planet and create a healthier environment for us all.

One of the most important ways that we can help to protect the global environment is by becoming more energy efficient in our homes and workplaces. The waste gases released into the atmosphere by the burning of fossil fuels, such as coal, gas, and oil, have a serious impact on the global climate and our health.

Burning fossil fuels produces so-called greenhouse gases, including carbon dioxide (CO_2). According to the Intergovernmental Panel on Climate Change, CO_2 emissions are the main cause of global warming. Greenhouse gases build up in the atmosphere, where they allow the sun's rays to warm the earth but prevent heat from escaping back into space—thus creating the greenhouse effect. This process is slowly but steadily increasing the earth's temperature.

Global warming has been blamed for meteorological disasters, such as hurricanes, floods, and droughts, and causing crop failures and disease. There is a very real threat that malaria could become common in Europe if temperatures rise any higher. And the melting of polar ice caps could cause flooding and other problems (see page 28).

GLOBAL CLIMATE CHANGE
Meteorological records show that global warming has been going on since the beginning of the industrial age. But scientific opinion is divided over whether humans are wholly responsible for this change or it is partly a natural phenomenon. The earth has warmed and cooled many times in its history, so the current changes may be part of a normal process. One thing is clear from a study of global weather patterns: an increase in the earth's average temperature eventually leads to dramatic changes in climate. Scientists who have studied the geological records of previous periods of warming on earth—some dating back thousands of years—say that the most dramatic changes in the global climate occur suddenly, leading to the extinction of some plant and animal species. Environmental groups believe that world governments should reduce greenhouse gas emissions now rather than wait for proof of the harm they might be causing. Otherwise, by the time the evidence becomes indisputable, climate changes may be irreversible.

At a climate change convention in Kyoto, Japan, in 1997, most industrial nations agreed to reduce emissions of greenhouse gases by 2012 to an average of 6 percent below 1990 levels. (The United States agreed to target 7 percent below its 1990 emission levels.) This can be achieved by energy-saving measures, such as making better use of nonpolluting forms of energy.

ACID RAIN

One of the most devastating effects that pollution has on the environment is acid rain. It has affected huge areas of forest land in both Europe and North American and has seriously damaged over 40 percent of the lakes in Sweden and 20 percent of the lakes in the United States. Acid rain is caused by sunlight acting on sulfur dioxide and nitrogen dioxide gases emitted by motor vehicles and coal-burning power plants. When combined with ozone and hydroxyl ions in the atmosphere and water in clouds, these gases form sulfuric acid and nitric acid, which fall as acid rain and snow.

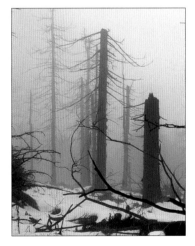

ACID ATTACK
The spruce trees in Karkonoski National Park in Poland have been devastated by acid rain; more than 3,700 acres have been damaged.

Origins

Until the 1950s the use of pesticides in farming was seen as wholly beneficial. Through the work of biologist Rachel Carson, however, the world began to realize the extensive dangers of uncontrolled chemical use in agriculture.

While working for the U.S. Fish and Wildlife Service in the 1930s and 1940s, Carson became aware that marine life was being harmed by modern farming practices. She alerted the world to the fact that pesticide residues were leaching from farmland into rivers, lakes, and the sea, causing extensive marine pollution. Her controversial 1962 book, *Silent Spring*, had the greatest impact, however. It warned that a build-up of pesticides such as DDT in the food chain would decimate wildlife and ultimately threaten the survival of humanity itself. The book led to stricter controls on pesticide use in agriculture.

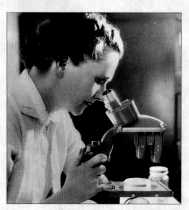

RACHEL CARSON (1907–1964)
Biologist Rachel Carson's book Silent Spring *warned of the apocalyptic consequences of uncontrolled pesticide use.*

The thinning ozone layer

Some man-made gases are damaging the ozone layer that protects the earth from the full impact of the sun's rays. While ozone may be harmful at ground level, it is highly beneficial in the upper atmosphere, where it filters out the damaging ultraviolet—UVB and UVC—rays from the sun. A reduced ozone layer means that we are at a higher risk for developing skin cancer.

The main threat to the ozone layer is posed by chlorofluorocarbons (CFCs), once used in aerosol cans, refrigerators, freezers, and some forms of packaging. Although most manufacturers have switched to safer gases, CFCs are still being released when discarded refrigerators are broken up for scrap.

To reduce the level of ozone-damaging gases, choose products labeled "ozone friendly" and have an old refrigerator or freezer disposed of by a company that salvages the gases and prevents them from being released into the environment. This is compulsory in the United States, with substantial fines for anyone caught not recycling refrigerant gases. Your local health department can give advice and information on how to dispose of your refrigerator or freezer in an environmentally friendly way.

The melting ice caps

One environmental change that has been directly linked to global warming is the melting of the polar ice caps. Temperatures in Antarctica have risen an average of 2.5°C (4.5°F) over the past 50 years. This has caused thousands of square miles of the polar ice shelf to break up and has increased the number of icebergs. Other polar changes include a rise in rainfall, a reduction in snow pack, and a ten-fold increase in the number of flowering plants. Patches of grass have even started to appear in Antarctica.

Ironically, some scientists fear that global warming may result in lower winter temperatures in northern Europe, particularly the United Kingdom. This is because of the effect it may have on the Gulf Stream. This huge current of warm water flows up from the Gulf of Mexico and bathes the British Isles and northern Europe in warm, moist air, keeping summer temperatures moderate and winter temperatures mild. Global changes, such as the release of freezing water from melting polar ice caps, may cause the Gulf Stream to change course, giving the United Kingdom a climate more like that in areas of Canada on the same latitude, with hot summers and arctic winters.

THE VANISHING FORESTS

Trees play a vital role in maintaining the equilibrium of the global environment, yet each year thousands of square miles of forest are lost. Much of this destruction provides wood for building and industry in the West. The United Kingdom alone uses more than 25 million cubic meters of lumber and lumber products each year. Ninety percent of this is imported from 50 different countries, many of which are losing their natural forests as a result. Every year 55,000 square miles of tropical forest are destroyed not only to provide lumber but also to create farmland. In the Philippines, for example, out of a total of 9,650 square miles of native forest, only 2,100 square miles are still adequately stocked. Other countries, including Brazil, Indonesia, Malaysia, Cameroon, and Ghana, are suffering similar problems.

Trees lower atmospheric levels of carbon dioxide by absorbing carbon and locking it into the structure of trunks and branches, often for hundreds of years. In the process oxygen is released, which is vital for all living creatures. When trees are burned or made into products that are later burned, carbon dioxide is released back into the atmosphere. Carbon dioxide levels can be kept in balance by planting more trees to replace those that are lost, but a better solution is to discourage the loss of trees in the first place.

Trees release into the air large quantities of water vapor that, in wooded areas, leads to cloud formation and rainfall and helps to prevent drought. Their root systems stabilize the ground, preventing soil erosion, which can lead to the spread of deserts and other environmental disasters. The devastating floods in Bangladesh in 1998 were widespread because of extensive deforestation in the region and in the nearby countries of India and Myanmar. A vast proportion of the country was under water, and millions of people were made homeless.

Forests are also home to a wide range of plant and animal species. They enhance the world's biodiversity—the variety of living species—helping to enrich our lives and to support the complex ecosystems of which

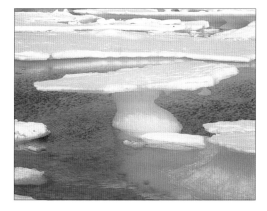

ANTARCTICA
Because of global warming, the temperature in Antarctica has risen, causing an increasing number of icebergs to break away from the polar ice shelf.

humankind is part. The trees most at risk from logging are tropical hardwoods (angiosperms), many of which are lovely but not necessarily durable. Some tropical hardwoods are harvested because they are cheap rather than because they are long-lasting. They come from tropical rain forests, and less than 0.2 percent are grown in a sustainable way. Their disappearance causes a loss of wildlife habitats, extinction of plants and animals, and soil erosion. The

THE EL NIÑO EFFECT

It has been suggested that global warming may increase the occurrences of El Niño, the current change that affects the West Coast of North America and many other regions. A huge current of warm water wells to the surface of the Pacific Ocean every three to seven years. Because it often appears at Christmas, it was named El Niño, or Christ child,

by Peruvian fishermen. The ecological repercussions can be devastating; populations of fish and other species can be wiped out, also destroying many livelihoods. El Niño's appearance in 1997 is thought to have been responsible for serious droughts in China and Australia, freak snow and ice storms in Canada, and an unprecedented 8 inches of snow in Jerusalem.

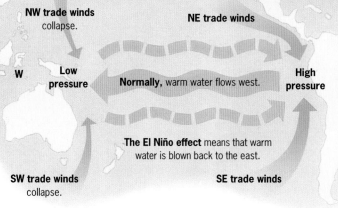

STORM DAMAGE
El Niño produces warm currents that change atmospheric pressure and completely reverse normal weather patterns. It has been blamed for such storms as Hurricane Hugo, which hit the East Coast of the United States in 1989, causing terrible damage.

EL NIÑO
Warm water normally runs west along the equator as a result of westerly trade winds caused naturally by the rotation of the earth. For reasons not fully understood, the winds reverse and blow eastward over the Pacific when El Niño occurs. This forces the warm water to flow eastward, affecting ocean temperatures on the west coast of South America.

NW trade winds collapse.

NE trade winds

W

Low pressure

Normally, warm water flows west.

High pressure

SW trade winds collapse.

The El Niño effect means that warm water is blown back to the east.

SE trade winds

associated logging and processing activities can cause pollution of natural water supplies. According to the International Tropical Timber Organization, over 300 species of tropical trees in Asia and Africa are under threat and some, including Brazilian rosewood and Chilean pine, are on the verge of extinction. Under the Convention on International Trade in Endangered Species (CITES), it is illegal to trade in endangered tropical hardwoods; species at risk but not endangered require permits.

Many softwood trees (gymnosperms) are grown on plantations in North America and Europe. They are managed in a sustainable way by planting more trees to replace those cut down. But plantations can still have an adverse environmental impact because natural forests are often cut down to make way for managed forests. Tree and plant species and much animal life may be lost in the process, as well as valuable habitats. About 80 percent of old-growth forests in the United States and 40 percent of Canada's original forests have already been lost, often to make way for commercial plantations.

SAVING THE FORESTS

Major reductions could be made in the amount of forest products imported by Western countries if wood products were used more efficiently and recycling efforts were improved. If you are buying tropical hardwood products, ask suppliers for written proof that the wood came from environmentally responsible and sustainable sources. The environmental campaign group Friends of the Earth will check the evidence to see whether it is genuine.

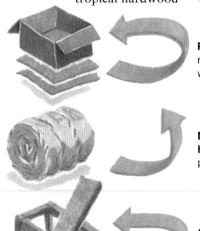

Paper and cardboard should be recycled. Buy recycled paper products whenever they are available.

Nonwood fibers, such as straw, grass, hemp, and flax, can be used for paper, particle board, and building materials.

Sound lumber from old furniture and house demolition should be reused rather than burned.

DEADLY SMOKE CLOUDS

In 1997 a program to cut down and burn about 2½ million acres of Indonesian rain forest to make way for rice paddies caused the world's worst man-made air pollution disaster. Smoke clouds from the resulting uncontrolled fires blanketed much of Southeast Asia and caused smoke pollution in cities at up to 7.5 milligrams of smoke particles per cubic meter of air. The previous record was set by a London smog in 1952 that reached 4.6 milligrams and led to 4,000 deaths.

THE TOXIC ENVIRONMENT

According to the U.S. National Institute of Environmental Health Sciences, people born since the 1940s face a two to three times greater risk of developing cancer than their parents and grandparents because of the increased level of agricultural and industrial chemicals in the environment. A study carried out by the institute in the mid-1990s linked the rise in cancers over the previous 50 years to the rapid rise in waste chemicals, many of which did not exist before. These include benzene, DDT, dioxin, and some additives in foods and drinks.

Of particular concern is exposure to the endocrine-disrupting chemicals contained in or released by the manufacture of plastics, detergents, pesticides, paint, ink, glue, some food packaging, and plastic toys. These are often discharged into rivers and lakes, where they become part of the food chain.

An endocrine disrupter is an agent that interferes with the normal production and/ or functions of natural hormones in the body. Attention has been focused especially on what are known as estrogenic chemicals, which act like estrogen in the body. It has been suggested that they may be causing a decline in sperm counts; a rise in reproductive abnormalities and disorders, such as undescended testicles and the gynecological condition endometriosis; and an increase in cancers of the testes, prostate, breasts, and ovaries. Research carried out independently in Britain, Denmark, and other countries suggests that sperm levels may have fallen by as much as 50 percent in many developed countries between 1940 and 1990.

FOOD CHAINS

The food chain is one of the main reasons that the destruction of habitats and the endangering of other species is of such concern to human well-being. We are part of a highly complicated and delicate balance of nature, and one small change in an ecosystem may create a massive effect, leading to threats to other species. Harmful chemicals used to treat the soil can infect the grass on which animals feed, the food crops grown in it, and the small animals that live in the soil. Pollution can affect humans more severely than many other animals because we are often at the end of a food chain and receive a larger, more harmful cocktail of toxins.

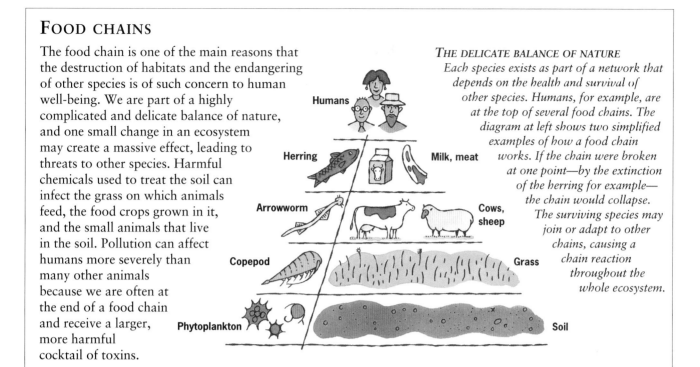

THE DELICATE BALANCE OF NATURE
Each species exists as part of a network that depends on the health and survival of other species. Humans, for example, are at the top of several food chains. The diagram at left shows two simplified examples of how a food chain works. If the chain were broken at one point—by the extinction of the herring for example— the chain would collapse. The surviving species may join or adapt to other chains, causing a chain reaction throughout the whole ecosystem.

Many estrogenic chemicals are lipophilic, or fat-loving, and thus are readily absorbed into fatty foods, such as dairy products and chocolates. They also accumulate in the fatty tissue of wildlife and humans. Such chemicals include phthalates, found in plastic containers and other forms of packaging.

Some scientists believe that the most damaging effect on health comes from chemicals called polychlorinated biphenyls (PCBs), which were a waste by-product of the plastics industry from the 1950s until banned in the 1970s. They are nonbiodegradable, which means they will exist in the environment indefinitely, and have been blamed for a rise in testicular cancer.

Sex changes in nature

The effects of chemical pollution on wildlife have been under scrutiny since the 1950s, thanks especially to the pioneering work of Rachel Carson. Further evidence emerged in the late 1980s, when zoologist Theodora Colborn discovered that contamination by hormonelike chemicals in the Great Lakes of North America had caused terrible reproductive abnormalities in 16 species of wildlife. Similar findings have been made in Massachusetts, Florida, and California.

In 1997 research carried out at Brunel University in England found that sewage pollution in eight English rivers had caused many fish to change sex. In two of these rivers, the Nene in Northamptonshire and the Aire in Yorkshire, all the roaches had developed both male and female characteristics. Female dogs along the British coastline have been found to develop male characteristics because of the use of tributyltin (TBT) as an antifouling agent.

The spread of toxic chemicals

Chemical pollution spreads all around the planet and contaminates even the most remote locations. Beluga and narwhal whales and polar bears have been found to contain high levels of insecticides, toxic metals such as mercury and cadmium, and industrial waste chemicals such as dioxin and PCBs. These pollutants come from thousands of miles away through a process called global distillation. They are drawn up into the atmosphere by evaporation and fall on northern regions in snow or rain. Further pollution by PCBs and DDT comes from highly contaminated Siberian rivers, which empty into the Arctic Ocean.

Native Inuit people, who live on wildlife like whales and seals, have high levels of toxins in their bodies. Over 16 percent of Greenland Inuits have potentially harmful levels of mercury in their blood, and breast-feeding Inuit mothers have five times the normal level of PCBs in their milk.

Overfishing

For thousands of years coastal communities have exploited the resources of the sea at a sustainable level. During the 20th century, however, the switch to intensive methods of fishing, such as drift nets and factory ships, seriously depleted fish stocks. In the 1970s overfishing almost wiped out herring in the North Atlantic and anchovies off the Peruvian coast. Overfishing can lead to enormous economic hardship, especially for the families and communities dependent on fish for food and/or income. The balance of the ocean ecosystem may also be disrupted, with major long-term consequences.

CARING FOR THE ENVIRONMENT

There is much you can do personally to create a healthier environment for everyone—from choosing ecologically friendly products to supporting green initiatives.

The problems facing the environment are too large for any one individual to combat, but there is plenty you can do to help prevent further deterioration of the natural world and preserve it for future generations. We all know that manufacturers and power plants produce much of the pollution that is affecting the atmosphere and that government and industry must adopt more policies that take environmental concerns into account. But domestic habits and lifestyles also have a profound effect. You can do your part by not contributing to pollution and by supporting those who are trying to reduce its impact and ensure that the planet remains healthy.

All societies must stop regarding the world's resources as something they have a right to exploit and take action to reduce destructive consequences. The planet's resources are limited; they should be used with care and with as little waste as possible.

Changing your own lifestyle in small ways can have a huge effect on the health of the environment. The more people there are who live responsibly, the more of an impact

they will have. A good starting point is to think and behave less materialistically. For example, you can repair items that you already own rather than purchase new ones, buy only products that you really need, and recycle as many things as possible.

Recycling
Recycling represents one of the most important ways that householders can support the environment. The throwaway culture that developed in the latter half of the 20th century led to a burgeoning problem with domestic waste. Fortunately, initiatives to turn this tide are paying off. The nation recycled or composted 27 percent of its municipal solid waste in 1995, up from 9.6 percent in 1980. But there is still a long way to go, and in recent times a few groups have emerged that oppose recycling.

In addition to saving energy and other resources, recycling reduces the need for incineration plants and landfill sites. Incinerators contribute to air pollution, and in densely populated areas landfill sites are a major problem. Not only are they an eyesore, but they also take up valuable space and blight the land for generations to come. Toxins leaching from landfill sites can con-

*CARING AND SHARING
Caring for the environment can be rewarding, satisfying, and fun. Joining an environmental action group can help you get to know fellow environmentalists and become involved with local issues.*

GREEN CHOICES

When shopping, try to choose products that have the least harmful impact on the environment. Look for items made from sustainable natural resources that do not contain potentially harmful ingredients. Minimal packaging lessens unnecessary waste. Below are examples of ecologically friendly and unfriendly products.

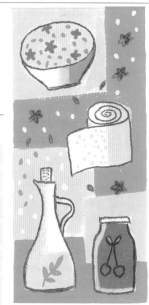

PRODUCT	ECO-FRIENDLY	ECO-UNFRIENDLY
Cotton balls, toilet paper	Unbleached, not dyed	Bleached, colored
Air fresheners	Potpourri, volcanic minerals	Aerosol
Deodorants	Roll-on	Aerosol
Household cleaners	Baking soda, vinegar	Many petroleum-based products
Milk containers	Reusable bottles	Cartons or plastic containers
Detergents	Phosphate-reduced, biodegradable	Many regular detergents

taminate underground water and poison rivers and streams. Another problem is that toxic gases emitted by landfills pollute the air and can build up to cause an explosion.

By law, all local authorities must have recycling systems in place and encourage the public to use them. It is now possible to recycle glass containers, certain types of plastic containers, aluminum and tin cans and other scrap metal, cardboard, and all kinds of paper, including newspapers, magazines, and catalogs. In addition, many communities are recycling garden clippings for mulch.

Many municipalities have recycled items picked up on a regular basis alongside the household trash. If yours does not and you must take your collection to a recycling site, try to avoid making special journeys and drop items off when you're making a trip that passes a recycling facility. Better still, encourage your local authority to install recycling bins near your home.

Many unwanted items can be given a new lease on life. Charities distribute donated items to people in need, and many run stores that sell unwanted items, such as clothing, books, toys, bric-a-brac, furniture, and music records and tapes. In addition to raising money for good causes, this form of recycling extends the life of these items and saves energy and resources. Yard sales and consignment shops offer additional opportunities for recycling items you have no further use for. Similarly, you can consider buying more secondhand clothing and other pre-owned items yourself rather than always purchasing new things. You can also recycle items more than once. For instance, you can use plastic or paper shopping bags for several trips to the supermarket, not just one or two; use both sides of paper; and reuse plastic tubs countless times before recycling them. There are many books available that suggest practical and creative ways to reuse all kinds of household items.

RECYCLING CORNER

One of the ways you can make recycling part of your daily routine is to set up recycling bins in convenient places around the house. For recycling food scraps to use as garden compost, keep containers right by the kitchen sink.

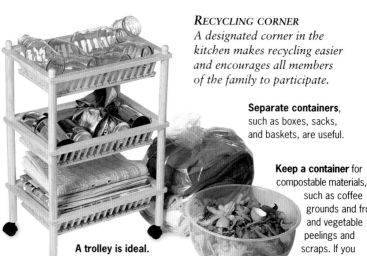

RECYCLING CORNER
A designated corner in the kitchen makes recycling easier and encourages all members of the family to participate.

Separate containers, such as boxes, sacks, and baskets, are useful.

Keep a container for compostable materials, such as coffee grounds and fruit and vegetable peelings and scraps. If you don't have a composter, you can bury them in your garden.

A trolley is ideal. Use separate levels for newspapers, bottles, cans, and charity items

Water quality

Water is under constant threat from contaminants, both natural and man-made. Although water companies treat water to make it as pure as possible, many people are still concerned about the safety of water in their home.

Without water, no life would be possible. Approximately 60 percent of an adult's body is composed of water. If too little water is consumed, serious health problems can result. Water is also vital for hygiene, to keep ourselves, our clothes, and our homes clean. However, water is also an efficient carrier of disease bacteria and other pollutants, so water purity and quality are very important issues.

Because safe drinking water is essential for health, it must meet high standards. The Environmental Protection Agency (EPA) sets the maximum contaminant level (MCL) for dozens of organic and inorganic

THE WATER CYCLE

Rainfall, our main source of water, can be affected by environmental factors. Sulfur dioxide and oxides of nitrogen in polluted air can dissolve in rainwater to make it highly acidic. It then falls as acid rain, often miles from where the pollution was produced.

THE WATER CYCLE
Water vapor rises from the earth into a cooler part of the atmosphere to form clouds. As the clouds rise, they cool further and give off water in the form of rain and snow.

Clouds are blown by the wind.

Clouds cool as they rise higher. Larger drops of water fall as rain or snow.

Rain

Transpiration: plants lose water through their leaves.

Clouds form as water vapor cools and condenses into tiny droplets of water.

Respiration: animals produce water vapor.

Water evaporates from bodies of water when warmed by the sun..

Water collects in streams.

Rivers flow into the sea.

Streams flow into rivers.

chemicals and several pathogens and radioactive pollutants that may be found in drinking water, and it monitors public water utilities to see that they meet these safe standards. Beaches and marinas in many areas also have to meet strict criteria for water quality (see page 155).

LEAD AND OTHER METALS

Lead is a toxin that affects the brain and nervous system. It has been recognized for centuries that high levels of lead in water could give rise to lead poisoning, but only fairly recently has its more subtle effects on health been identified, especially its potential to lower the IQ in children. Evidence has also emerged that low levels of lead may raise blood pressure in some adults.

Water leaving a treatment plant is virtually lead free, but it can become contaminated with lead in your home plumbing or the pipes that connect your home to the water service. Homes built in this country before 1930 were usually fitted with lead pipes. (Unpainted lead pipes are dull gray and quite soft; scraping gently with a knife will reveal shiny, silver-colored metal.) Those built or renovated between 1930 and 1986 are likely to have copper pipes with lead soldering. Since 1986 regulations have required all new buildings to have lead-free pipe and solder.

Lead from pipes may dissolve in water, particularly soft water. In hard-water regions a buildup of lime scale tends to coat the lead and prevent it from dissolving.

If you believe you may have lead in your plumbing, there are a few simple precautions you can take. Use only cold water for drinking and cooking and run the tap for several minutes before using the water if it has been standing in the pipes overnight or for several hours during the day. You can also have your water tested, a good idea especially if you draw it from a well. The MCL for lead is 15 parts per billion (ppb). If your

water exceeds this level, there are some measures that will correct the problem. You can install a corrosion control device where your water enters your plumbing system; have your plumbing replaced with plastic pipes or copper pipes joined with lead-free solder; or install a ceramic filter at the kitchen sink for cooking and drinking water. You may want to consult an expert before deciding which is the best option for you.

Other metals likely to be found in drinking water include copper and aluminum. Copper comes from domestic water pipes and seldom causes health problems, although it may discolor toilets, tubs, and sinks if levels are high. When the water has not been used for a long period, it is advisable to allow the tap to run for several minutes to draw in fresh water from the water main.

Aluminum is found naturally in water and is also used often in water treatment systems to help remove particles, including microorganisms. At one time there was concern about a possible link between aluminum and Alzheimer's disease, but after much research most experts believe this to be very unlikely. Drinking water standards prevent aluminum from settling in the public water main and causing dirty water.

Arsenic, a toxic metallic element, also occurs naturally in water, but it is a product of industrial and agricultural waste too, particularly insecticides. The present standard is a maximum of 50 parts per billion, but many experts believe it should be as little as 3 ppb, and the EPA is now suggesting that the allowable level be changed to 5 ppb. Arsenic in drinking water can cause bladder, lung, and skin cancer and possibly liver and kidney cancer. It damages the nervous system and heart and blood vessels as well.

To reduce exposure to harmful metals in water, do not use hot water from the faucet to fill a kettle or to drink and particularly not to prepare

Water is pumped from a river or lake and stored in a reservoir.

At the purifying plant lumps of solid matter settle to the bottom of the sedimentation tank.

Sand beds filter out small particles.

Chlorine is added to kill germs.

The pumping station pumps clean water to users.

When the tap is turned on, safe drinking water flows out of it.

FROM THE LAKES TO THE TAPS
The water in a public system is taken from lakes and rivers. Before it comes out of our taps, it goes through purifying treatments to make it safe to drink.

a baby's formula. Hot water leaches far more minerals from pipes than cold water does.

Fluoride

Fluoride is found naturally in many water sources. It offers protection against tooth decay, but if levels rise above the drinking water standard of 1.5 mg per liter, there is an increased risk of a condition called dental fluorosis—discoloration, mottling, and pitting of teeth. Very high concentrations can result in a crippling brittle-bone condition called skeletal fluorosis. If fluoride levels are found to be above the maximum standard, such water is usually blended with low-fluoride water to reduce the concentration.

For years the addition of fluoride to water supplies has been recommended by many dental health authorities and the World Health Organization (WHO). A great deal of evidence indicates that the current recommended level is safe, but there is considerable controversy today over just how beneficial fluoride is, if at all, and many groups are fighting to keep it out of public systems.

Microbiological quality

Many microorganisms that cause disease can be carried in water. The most serious diseases, such as cholera and typhoid, are largely under control in developed countries, but outbreaks of illness can still occur when water treatment controls are breached. One concern is a gastrointestinal parasite called cryptosporidium, which is excreted from infected animals and humans as oocysts and causes severe diarrhea. Cryptosporidium can be contracted in various ways, but a number of waterborne outbreaks have been identified. Most of these resulted from problems with the filtration process during water treatment, which normally removes the oocysts that are resistant to chlorination. There is a major worldwide research program aimed at finding new ways of combating these organisms.

Nitrates

Nitrates can be a problem in both surface and ground water. The main source in soil is nitrogen from artificial fertilizers or animal waste that is not taken up by plants. The excess is washed out of the soil by rainwater and carried into rivers and lakes. The WHO standard for nitrates, 50 mg per liter of water, aims at preventing a condition called blue-baby syndrome, which occurs in bottle-fed infants up to about three months of age. Claims have also been made that nitrates in water are linked with reproductive and developmental defects and cancer, but the evidence remains inconclusive.

Wetlands that contain cattails and reeds have been found to absorb many pollutants, including nitrogen, phosphorus, and heavy metals that are toxic to humans. Reed beds are now being used by many municipalities to purify groundwater.

Pesticides

At least 22 pesticides have been identified in well water in this country. Levels of safety have been set for many of them, but the fact is that the long-term effects of most pesticides have not been determined.

Herbicides are another problem. Because they are more water soluble and mobile than insecticides, they are more likely to get into water supplies. Those most often detected in drinking water are isoproturon, atrazine, simazine, chlortoluron, and diuron. When herbicides are found in public water supplies, they rarely exceed EPA guidelines. However, there is little information on the levels in private water supplies in agricultural areas. Atrazine and simazine can no longer be used in areas where they may contaminate water, and so their frequency of detection in drinking water is falling. For other herbicides, such as isoproturon, that can be long-term contaminants, farmers are being encouraged to develop better practices to prevent toxic chemicals from reaching drinking water supplies.

Chlorine

Used as a disinfectant for drinking water for nearly a century, chlorine has contributed to the eradication of several serious waterborne diseases in many parts of the world. However, it can react with naturally occurring organic matter in the water to produce a number of unwanted by-products, such as

---

PROTECTING TEETH FROM DECAY

A fluoride level in drinking water of about 1 mg per liter helps to protect children's teeth from dental decay. Municipalities that have this optimum concentration show better dental health than those with a similar socioeconomic profile and lower fluoride levels. Above the optimum level, however, there are serious health risks.

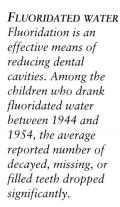

FLUORIDATED WATER Fluoridation is an effective means of reducing dental cavities. Among the children who drank fluoridated water between 1944 and 1954, the average reported number of decayed, missing, or filled teeth dropped significantly.

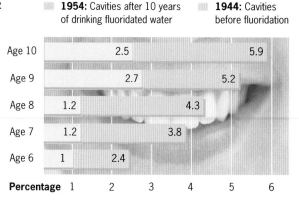

1954: Cavities after 10 years of drinking fluoridated water

1944: Cavities before fluoridation

Age	1954	1944
Age 10	2.5	5.9
Age 9	2.7	5.2
Age 8	1.2	4.3
Age 7	1.2	3.8
Age 6	1	2.4

Percentage 1 2 3 4 5 6

chloroform and trihalomethanes, which are known to be carcinogenic. Although levels of chlorine are lower than in the past, studies are ongoing to determine other adverse effects that might be associated with it. This research reflects the need to strike a balance between the benefits of chlorine in destroying microorganisms and the effects of long-term exposure.

IMPROVING WATER SUPPLIES

Many people prefer not to use water straight from the municipal supply. Some dislike the taste of chlorine; others are concerned about possible contamination by microorganisms and chemicals. Whatever the reason, there are various alternatives.

Water treatment in the home

There are two basic types of water treatment systems for the home; one kind is installed where water enters the house, the other where water is used, such as the kitchen sink. The price and effectiveness of systems vary considerably. A nonprofit organization, NSF International, certifies water treatment devices that perform as claimed. Whatever device you choose, it must be operated and maintained according to the instructions to be effective.

Filter systems may contain activated carbon, which can remove organic compounds and pesticides; a ceramic filter, which removes inorganic chemicals, dirt particles, rust, and heavy metals such as lead; or an ultraviolet (UV) filter, which kills viruses, an important consideration for anyone whose immune system is weakened. Some household units contain all three types of filter and come in models that fit under the counter or on the countertop. It is important to find out which contaminants are present in your household water in order to select the most suitable type of filter.

In hard-water areas, a deionizer, or water softener, can significantly reduce the buildup of scale in water

pipes and improve the effectiveness of detergents and soaps for washing. However, it is recommended that the pipe supplying drinking water not be connected to the softener because deionized water often contains high levels of sodium, which can be detrimental for bottle-fed infants and people on low-sodium diets, such as those who have high blood pressure. (Using potassium chloride instead of sodium chloride in the system can get around this problem.)

A water-distilling system may be the most effective of all. It removes bacteria, viruses, cysts, heavy metals, particulates, radionuclides, volatile organic compounds, and minerals. Water distillers are expensive, about 25 cents per gallon on average, but cost less than bottled water.

Bottled water

Bottled water can be a very convenient but expensive alternative to tap water. If purchased because of concerns about the safety of tap water, bottled waters do not always represent good value because some also contain contaminants. Bottled waters are monitored but perhaps not as strictly as they should be. There is a bewildering array of brands, and the source is not always indicated. By law, only water from natural sources, such as underground springs, can be called "natural mineral water." Others are taken from municipal supplies and then carbonated and/or flavored.

Conserving water

Water shortages have increased in many parts of the country, resulting in part from less rainfall but also from a rise in demand. Although efforts are

WATER USAGE
The average household uses about 35 gallons of water per day for activities like washing dishes and taking showers. Up to 4½ gallons can be wasted daily through dripping taps and leaking pipes.

being made to reduce leakage from water distribution systems, combating the problem will require much more effort. There are many water conservation measures that you can use in the home and garden. Washing the car, for example, does not require water of drinking standard. Reusing water from baths and washing machines (called gray water) is a useful option, especially when supplies are scarce. Some companies offer systems for collecting water so that it can be reused conveniently; these are fairly expensive, however.

Watering a garden puts a high demand on the water supply; this can be reduced by watering in the morning to minimize evaporation, installing a drip system, and planting drought-tolerant species.

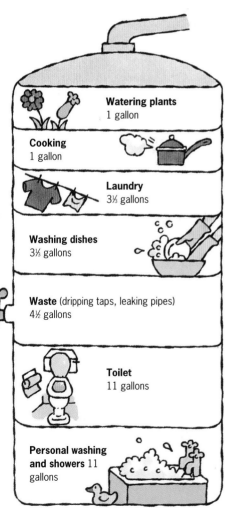

Watering plants
1 gallon

Cooking
1 gallon

Laundry
3¼ gallons

Washing dishes
3¼ gallons

Waste (dripping taps, leaking pipes)
4½ gallons

Toilet
11 gallons

Personal washing and showers 11 gallons

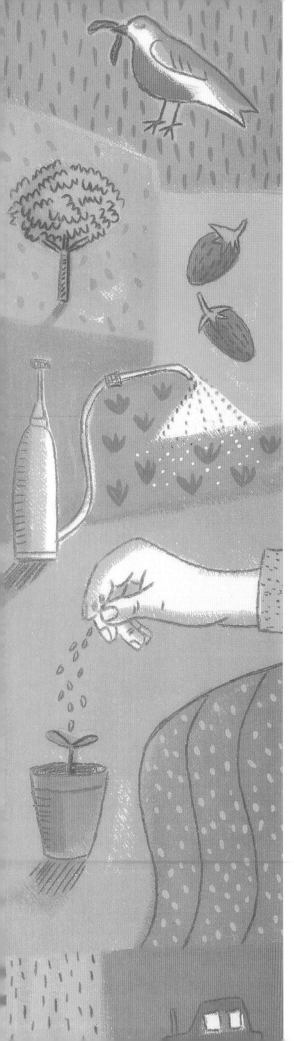

Saving the soil

Healthy soil is vital for a healthy planet, yet it is increasingly under threat from being washed or blown away, contaminated, and depleted of nutrients. Some farmers are returning to traditional agriculture methods to protect the soil for the future.

Soil literally holds the ecosystem together. It provides stability and essential nutrients for plants and homes for countless animals, and it is the very basis of the agriculture upon which we depend for our food. Indeed, some of the nutrients we obtain from plants, such as the antioxidant selenium, are present in vegetables solely because of the soil in which they are grown.

Some soil erosion is natural and is rectified by new soil being created all the time from underlying bedrock and decaying animal and vegetable matter. Erosion becomes a problem when it takes place faster than new soil can form. If this happens, the land becomes less fertile and can turn eventually into desert, a process known as desertification. Today desertification is affecting more than 100 countries. A global survey by the International Soil Reference and Information Center calculated that 22 million acres of land are extremely degraded and 3 billion acres—about 10 percent of the earth's vegetation-covered surface— are at least moderately degraded.

PREVENTING SOIL EROSION

The top few centimeters of soil contain the most nutrients. This topsoil can easily be blown or washed away by wind and rain, leading to poor soil and weak plants that are prone to disease.

HEALTHY SOIL
Many steps can be taken to reduce topsoil erosion and ensure the growth of healthy plants.

Tree and grass roots help to hold the soil in place.

Hedges act as a wind barrier and reduce the loss of topsoil.

Plowing so that furrows lie across the natural slope of the land prevents rainwater from running down the furrows and washing the soil away.

A terraced hillside slows down the flow of rain and allows it to soak into the soil to nourish crops.

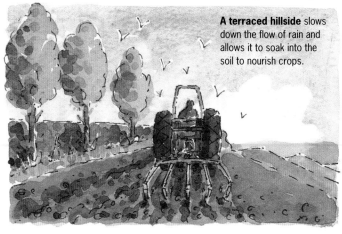

CAUSES OF SOIL EROSION

Vegetation protects the soil from erosion, so conditions can quickly deteriorate if shrubs and plants are removed—for example, by plowing or felling trees. Without vegetation topsoil can be washed away by rainwater or blown away by winds. Salination also increases erosion. High salt concentrations can result from poorly designed irrigation systems, excessive withdrawal of groundwater in coastal areas, or infiltration by seawater.

Bad farm management is the underlying cause of vegetation loss and is thought to be damaging an area equal to 38 percent of cropland worldwide. Physical deterioration of land is also a significant factor; it can be caused by compaction (with heavy machinery), waterlogging, or natural settling.

Fertilizers and pesticides

Even where the soil remains in place, it may deteriorate in quality as a result of contamination. The most important impact has come from the use of artificial fertilizers and pesticides—collectively known as agrochemicals. Artificial fertilizers are compounds used to put nutrients back into the soil and restore its fertility. Nitrate, added to supply nitrogen—an essential nutrient for plant growth—is often a component.

Modern farming practices have resulted in dramatic increases in the use of fertilizers. In 1996 global use reached 116 million tons—a staggering rise from just 13 million tons in 1950. As a result, there are now much higher levels of fertilizer residues in many soils. Using too many fertilizers or applying them in the wrong place causes problems. Some residues leach into rivers and groundwater aquifers, where they cause pollution. Others are stored in the plants that they help to grow; for example, lettuces grown in winter can build up unnaturally high levels of nitrate in their leaves.

The use of pesticides is even more worrying. Pesticides are harmful not just to weeds, pests, and fungi; most are also capable of damaging other species. Global pesticide sales are growing at nearly 2 percent a year, the largest growth occurring in Africa, Asia, and Latin America. These chemicals may also get into the food chain, where they intensify in their effect. The use of pesticides inspired Rachel Carson's groundbreaking 1962 book, *Silent Spring,* which warned how these toxic substances were harming animals, such as birds and rodents, by contaminating their food.

Pesticides enter the soil in a variety of ways—through overspraying, the runoff from spraying or accidental spillage; in the feces of exposed animals; and as a result of treated organisms being incorporated into the soil. They can have a highly detrimental effect on the soil ecosystem, including soil respiration and soil organisms.

GLOBAL FERTILIZER USE

The increasing use of synthetic fertilizers is shown here in kilograms per hectare (2.47 acres). Excessive levels of fertilizer can harm the earth's ecosystem.

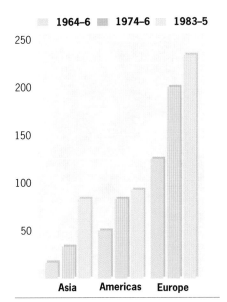

| 1964–6 | 1974–6 | 1983–5 |

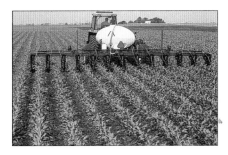

SYNTHETIC FERTILIZERS
A tractor applies a chemical solution containing nitrogen to a field of young corn plants. While synthetic fertilizers do help rebalance depleted soils, artificially high levels of nitrogen can build up in crops that grow in the treated soil.

Earthworms are important animals that reside in the soil. They help to maintain soil structure and fertility by burrowing holes and dragging down nutritious vegetation from the surface. They also interact with plant roots and soil microorganisms and provide a vital food source for birds and invertebrate predators. Yet pesticide residues are regularly killing these and other soil creatures.

Deprived of living organisms, the soil becomes less fertile and able to support life. In a vicious spiral the use of agrochemicals often leads to the use of more agrochemicals to put right the unexpected side effects of previous applications. Effects can be of long duration, particularly with the longer-lasting chemicals. Organophosphate and organochlorine insecticides can persist in the soil for more than 15 years and can build up to harmful levels in the bodies of soil animals.

Chemical waste

It would be unfair to blame soil contamination entirely on the farmer. In Europe alone, more than 35 million acres of land are contaminated with industrial and urban waste, particularly, but not only, in the former Eastern Bloc countries. Soil degradation can be caused by several factors, including acid rain and mining, as well as

SOIL ORGANISMS AND CHEMICAL WASTE

Millions of organisms live in the soil, and all have essential roles in the nutrient cycle, ensuring healthy soil and thus the growth of healthy plants for food. Bacteria and fungi are important for decomposing dead organic materials, while worms maintain soil structure and fertility. Fertilizers and pesticides may kill such organisms and contaminate the soil, which then becomes poorer and unable to sustain life. This causes the food for birds and animals to be reduced or contaminated and may lead to long-term problems.

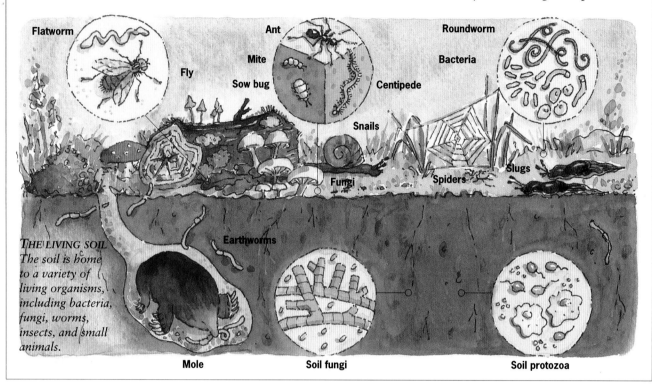

Flatworm · Ant · Mite · Fly · Sow bug · Roundworm · Bacteria · Centipede · Snails · Fungi · Spiders · Slugs

THE LIVING SOIL
The soil is home to a variety of living organisms, including bacteria, fungi, worms, insects, and small animals.

Mole · Earthworms · Soil fungi · Soil protozoa

industrial, residential, and agricultural waste. In Poland, for example, levels of lead and cadmium in the soil around Olkusz and Slawkow are the highest ever recorded in the world. Although Poland has the highest concentration of heavy industry in Europe, 50 percent of the land there is still used for agriculture or urban garden allotments, and 40 percent of all locally consumed vegetables and fruits are grown in the region.

According to the World Health Organization (WHO), 60 to 80 percent of heavy metals enter the human body through food. Some Polish experts have called for a ban on the consumption of food grown in areas contaminated with heavy metals, pesticides, and excessive nitrates.

Effects on food

Recently there has been growing concern about pesticide levels in food because monitoring programs continue to reveal high levels of residues. In 1995 the results of U.K. research into the levels of organophosphates and carbamate residues in carrot roots revealed that 1 to 2 percent of carrots contained 25 times more than expected. In other countries, such as China and some parts of Africa, the figure is higher.

Problems are compounded by the presence of occasional peaks of residue pollution. The WHO assesses acceptable daily intakes (ADIs) for a range of toxic chemicals. These ADIs are based on lifetime exposure through normal consumption of the crops containing those residue levels. The findings from the U.K. research

on carrots showed that the ADI was exceeded by up to three times in half of the carrots tested. The results from this research prompted studies by the Advisory Committee on Pesticides into pesticide residues in other produce. The first year's results found similar variability in other crops; the highest occurred in nectarines, which revealed organophosphate levels exceeding the average by up to 29 times.

Researchers in New Zealand in the 1990s reported pesticide residues in 56 percent of the food samples analyzed. The level of fungicide residues was more than 13 times higher than in similar foods grown in the United States.

Similar results have been found for fertilizers. As levels of nitrate in the environment have increased, so have the levels in food, particularly vegetables. Plants take up nitrate through their roots, and if it is not used immediately for the synthesis of amino acids and nucleic acids, it is stored in the cells. Concentrations increase with heavy use of fertilizers. Each part of a plant stores a different amount of nitrate. As a rule, stem and leaf tissues accumulate the most, followed by roots and lastly flowers and fruit. Nitrate levels can vary enormously among species and within any given type of vegetable.

Crops that can build up high nitrate levels are beets and leafy vegetables, such as spinach, lettuce, and cabbage. Research also suggests that some modern varieties tend to accumulate higher nitrate levels than traditional ones. Modern crops, which are bred for maximum yield, build up large reserves of nitrate within their cells, and these can still be present at harvest.

Prevention measures
Around the world more people are facing up to the challenge of discovering—or rediscovering—effective ways of using the soil in order to maintain quality. Thousands of projects are underway to address the problem of soil erosion and degradation, and a United Nations Convention on Drought and Desertification is coordinating an international response. The primary task is to reintroduce vegetation to areas where it has been lost, which will help to stabilize the soil and in time change local weather patterns and ultimately provide a richer, more balanced ecology.

Elsewhere the question of chemical waste is being addressed, although the problem is equally huge because once soil is contaminated, it can remain so for a long time. Changes in industrial practices, improved waste treatment, and enforcement of existing regulations can all help to reduce contamination. Other help is available from plants found to

absorb chemical contaminants from the soil; one example is fescue grass, which removes petroleum waste.

Many farmers are seeking solutions to declining soil fertility because they suffer directly from falling yields and the need for a higher input of fertilizer. Some are looking at better methods of application, safer pesticides that quickly break down into harmless by-products, and slow-release fertilizers to help encourage soil life. A growing number are turning their backs on agrochemicals altogether and choosing to farm organically.

The International Federation of Organic Agriculture Movements (IFOAM) defines organic agriculture as systems that take "soil fertility as a key to successful production by dramatically reducing chemical and genetically synthesized fertilizers, pesticides, and pharmaceuticals." Organic farmers rely on crop rotation, natural fertilizers, use of nitrogen-fixing plants like legumes, and natural predators to control pests.

Twenty years ago farmers using such approaches were written off as unrealistic amateurs or utopians. Today organic food is a multi-million-dollar business showing a healthy growth. There are more than 500 organic organizations in the IFOAM from virtually every corner of the world. Putting soil back at the center of agriculture is proving attractive to an ever-increasing number of farmers.

Improving soil quality
To help improve the overall quality of soil, you as an individual can buy organic food, which should be certified organic by a local authority. While this measure is no guarantee that food is totally uncontaminated (pesticides can drift in the wind, and soil can remain contaminated for decades), it does reduce the chances of contamination. You can also improve soil quality in your own garden by using organic methods. Many catalogs and nurseries offer products that make the task easy.

CROP ROTATION

Organic farmers use a system called crop rotation. This involves varying the types of crops that are grown in particular fields so that the same crop is not grown in the same place in successive years. Some crops remove nutrients from the soil, while others put them back. Rotating crops ensures that the soil stays naturally rich in nutrients, and it also slows down the rate of soil degeneration, thus reducing the need for pesticides and fertilizers.

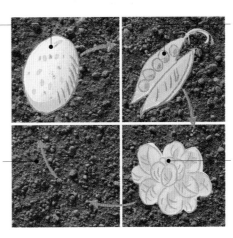

Root vegetables are nutrient-hungry crops. Because the soil has been fully enriched during the rest period, the crop can be grown successfully.

Peas and beans put nitrogen into the soil.

An unplanted plot allows soil time to recover, during which it can be enriched with organic matter.

Leafy vegetables are nitrogen-hungry crops.

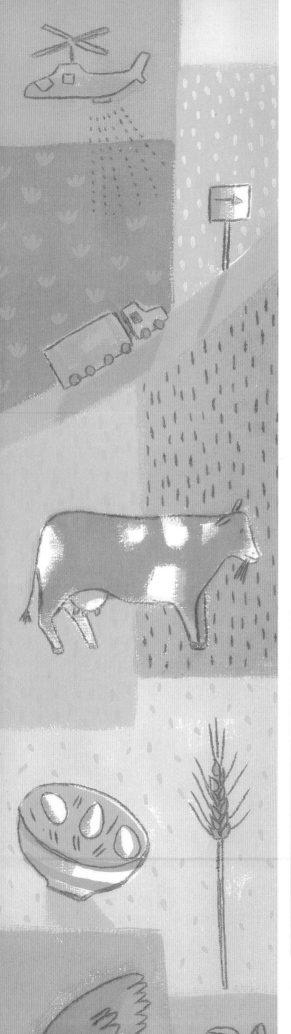

Food

Modern intensive farming is so productive that some countries now have a problem with food surpluses rather than shortages. However, this success has led to other concerns that must be tackled, such as chemical and bacterial contamination.

As medical scientists discover new links between diet and health, the old adage "You are what you eat" has never seemed more appropriate. On average most Westerners have eaten 27 tons of food by the age of 70. Yet the way that much modern food is produced, with its reliance on chemical sprays, intensive raising systems for farm animals, and a battery of additives, has led many to question the safety of today's food.

Well-publicized cases of *E. coli* and salmonella food poisoning have focused attention on the way that food is produced and handled, while reports of contaminants in food from pesticides, certain additives, and food packaging has led to a search for more environmentally friendly products by consumers.

AGROCHEMICALS

Modern farming has become more reliant on the intensive use of pesticides and fertilizers to protect plants against pests and diseases and to boost crop production. In addition to killing insects, weeds, fungi, and molds, agrochemicals are sometimes used after harvesting to prevent food from deteriorating during storage or transportation.

The public is exposed to pesticides and other chemicals largely through the food and water they consume,

CHILDREN AND PESTICIDES

Whatever the risks to adults from pesticide residues, children are often more at risk. This is because in relation to their weight children consume more food than adults, they are developing more rapidly, especially their brains and nervous systems, and their bodies are less efficient at getting rid of toxins. In 1989 the U.S. Natural Resources Defense Council revealed that at least 17 percent of preschool children were exposed to toxic organophosphate insecticides from fruits and vegetables at levels above those considered safe by the Environmental Protection Agency.

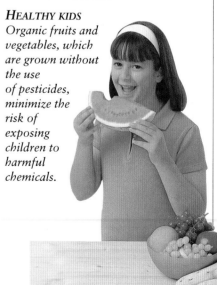

HEALTHY KIDS
Organic fruits and vegetables, which are grown without the use of pesticides, minimize the risk of exposing children to harmful chemicals.

which may contain chemical residues. There have been a few cases of direct pesticide poisoning, but occupational exposure—for example, through spraying on farms—is more common. Many farmers claim that the organophosphate insecticides used in sheep dips cause debilitating health effects, including impaired mental function and chronic nerve damage.

Incidences of accidental pesticide poisoning are rare in developed countries, although they do happen. One of the worst cases occurred in 1985 when several hundred people in the United States suffered severe stomach pains after eating watermelons contaminated with the pesticide aldicarb. The chemical probably entered through water used on the fruit. In 1995 the U.K. Ministry of Agriculture, Fisheries, and Food warned that eating carrots could cause stomach pains as a result of the organophosphate pesticides used to treat carrot fly.

A concern for many people is the possible health risk from a lifetime of exposure to minute amounts of pesticide residues in food and drinking water. Pesticides are designed to be toxic. In tests on laboratory animals, nearly 40 percent of the 400 or so chemicals used as pesticides were found, in very large doses, to cause cancer, reproductive disorders such as impotency and birth defects, and genetic mutations.

DDT was developed in 1939 as a solution to epidemics worldwide, such as the typhus spread by lice in Naples in 1943. When it was introduced, DDT was heralded as a savior that would eradicate all pests that carry diseases, but it has since been banned in many countries. It does not break down easily and becomes increasingly concentrated in the food chain until it reaches potentially harmful levels in animals that are higher up the chain, such as birds, mammals, and eventually humans (see box above).

PESTICIDES AND THE FOOD CHAIN

When pesticides are used to clear water supplies of bacteria or insects, they can have great effects on the ecology of the area. In the 1950s in Clear Lake, California, DDT was sprayed to control mosquitoes, which carry disease. However, the pesticide became lodged in the water, which then contaminated the plant and pond life, killing all the local birds that fed from the lake.

DEADLY CHAIN OF EVENTS
Pesticides infect water and intensify at each step in the food chain, resulting in a lethal cocktail of chemicals.

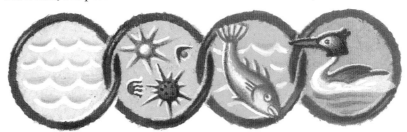

Water: 0.02 ppm of DDT   **Plankton:** 5 ppm of DDT   **Fish:** 250 ppm of DDT   **Grebes:** 1600 ppm of DDT—possibly lethal

The impact on humans of much smaller levels of exposure over a longer period of time is still largely unknown. A 1990 report by the British Medical Association concluded that "we do not know whether pesticides are harmful or not in day-to-day use. Until we have a more complete understanding of pesticide toxicity, the benefit of the doubt should be awarded to protecting the environment, the worker, and the consumer."

There are fears that higher-than-average rates of breast cancer in some areas where farming is intensive may be linked to pesticide use, and some researchers believe that certain people may be sensitive to even minute amounts of pesticide residues and suffer such reactions as migraine, abdominal pain, asthma, and eczema. There have also been suggestions that chronic fatigue syndrome may result from pesticide exposure. Health officials maintain that all pesticides licensed for use are rigorously tested and safe when used as directed, and while small amounts of pesticide residues may turn up in food, these are usually within safe levels. Yet this is not always the case.

In Great Britain 1 to 2 percent of fruits and vegetables sampled by government tests exceed permitted maximum residue levels (MRLs), while in the United States the Food and Drug Administration has reported that 10 percent of food imported into the country contains illegal levels of detectable pesticides. Some of the most toxic and persistent pesticides, such as DDT, have been banned in the developed world, yet many of these pesticides are still being used in developing countries and can return as residues in imported food.

Although actual risks from pesticide residues may be small, the perceived risk by individuals is often greater. Pesticide residues cannot be seen and in many cases cannot be washed off, so individuals are often unsure about the risk they are taking. Many people are now choosing to buy organic produce, which is grown without the use of chemical sprays and fertilizers. This not only minimizes possible risks to their own and their children's health but also supports a form of agriculture that is less harmful to the environment and wildlife.

GENETICALLY ENGINEERED FOOD

Biotechnology companies have been investing huge sums into developing genetically engineered plants, and these are now used in many processed foods. Genetic technology enables scientists to alter the gene structure of plants and animals and create varieties that are disease or pest resistant, have a longer shelf life, or are more appealing. Supporters claim they are simply speeding up a process pursued for centuries through selective crossbreeding and that benefits include increased yield and reduced need for pesticides and fertilizers. Critics argue that selective breeding cannot cross the species barrier as genetic modification does, for instance, by introducing a fish gene into a tomato to achieve a desired effect. Furthermore, they argue, genetically modified organisms (GMOs) might cross-pollinate with wild plants to produce superweeds, and insecticide-resistant plants might destroy beneficial insects, eventually affecting the food chain. More research is needed to understand the long-term consequences of GMOs, and there are increasing demands for the labeling of foods that contain them so that choice rests with the consumer.

Sex-change chemicals

It is now known that many of the chemicals released into the environment can interfere with the normal development and functioning of hormones in animals, including humans; one in particular mimics the female hormone estrogen. These chemicals, known as endocrine disrupters, have been dubbed gender-benders because they may be responsible for sex changes observed in wildlife. They include pesticides and some chemicals used in plastics and detergents. Their effects on humans at a low level of exposure are still unclear, but a number of scientists believe they may be linked to declining sperm counts in men, reproductive and sexual development disorders, reduced fertility, and even certain cancers (see page 30).

Hormones

Hormones have for years been fed to animals as growth enhancers. Some, such as steroids, are permitted in meat production in the United States but are currently banned in Europe, although traces of illegal growth promoters, such as clenbuterol, sometimes turn up in meat there.

Tests found a small amount of steak and beef liver in the United Kingdom to be contaminated with minute, probably harmless doses of illegal growth promoters, but far less than found in some other European countries. In Spain clenbuterol in beef is known to have caused several deaths.

Antibiotics are routinely added to the feed of intensively raised farm animals to quicken their growth and prevent weight-loss infections that are rife in overcrowded conditions. Traces of residues from these drugs can turn up in milk, meat, and farmed fish, and there is concern that their use is encouraging the growth of drug-resistant superbugs that are affecting human health.

Vitamin A, which is stored naturally in the liver, is also used as a growth promoter, and excess levels have been found in the liver of animals. Pregnant women are advised to avoid eating liver because too high concentrations of vitamin A can harm an unborn baby.

Additives

The additives used in food include colorings, preservatives, artificial sweeteners and other flavor enhancers, emulsifiers, thickeners (to enhance consistency), and vitamins and minerals (to improve or maintain nutritive value). They allow people to enjoy a wide variety of unspoiled and flavorful food year-round without the inconvenience of shopping every day.

The Food and Drug Administration (FDA) is responsible for approving all food additives used in the United States and for defining the truthful labeling of ingredients. A manufacturer must prove an additive's safety to the FDA before it can be used, and once approved, it is designated GRAS, or "generally recognized as safe." Even package materials must be approved by the FDA because trace amounts can leach into food during storage.

To help serve as an ongoing safety check of all additives, the FDA also operates the Adverse Reaction Monitoring System (ARMS). This agency investigates complaints from individuals or their doctors that seem to be related to specific foods. A number of additives appear to cause asthma, rashes, or other allergic reactions in people who are sensitive to them. When quite a few such reactions have been reported, the ARMS must decide whether they represent enough of a public health hazard that the additive should be banned for use.

There has also been concern that additives might cause hyperactivity in children. However, the true incidence of such reactions to additives is now found to be lower than was originally thought. A small percentage of children can react to synthetic food colorings and a few preservatives, while others may be sensitive to naturally occurring ingredients, such as salicylates, which are found in certain fruits and vegetables.

Some additives have been linked to cancers, reproductive problems, and other disorders in laboratory test animals, yet the effects on humans of amounts generally consumed in the diet over a long period are not known. Margins of safety are built into permitted levels of use, but there is an inherent uncertainty in applying the results on experimental rats to humans. In addition, the possible synergistic, or cocktail, effect of a mixture of additives in the body cannot be fully assessed.

FOOD CONTAMINANTS

Potentially toxic substances can enter the body through food. The most dangerous of these are aflatoxins—toxic chemicals produced by a mold that grows on peanuts, Brazil nuts, pistachio nuts, and dried figs—which can cause liver damage and cancer.

Aluminum from saucepans, beverage containers, and food wrappings can pass into acidic foodstuffs, and at one time a link was suspected between aluminum consumption and Alzheimer's disease. Research so far has not confirmed this possibility.

Bisphenol A, which is used to coat the inside of tin cans and bottle tops, can leach into vegetables. It mimics estrogen in the body and is therefore

an endocrine disrupter (see "Sex-change chemicals," opposite page).

Lead can be absorbed by crops grown near roads or industrial plants or land that contains high levels of industrial waste. It accumulates in the body; babies and young children are most at risk because lead can retard intellectual development.

Another possible, though rare contaminant is ochratoxin A, a toxin produced by a mold found mainly on cereal, coffee, cocoa, figs, and nuts; it can cause kidney disease.

The most effective way to avoid toxic substances in food is to buy fresh produce from a reputable supermarket or greengrocer, avoid eating moldy products, and store food correctly (see below).

Effects of food on pollution

The way in which food is produced and distributed can have an impact on health in less direct ways. Much of modern agriculture is dependent on nonrenewable sources of energy, such as oil- and coal-based fuels, and a very high level of energy is consumed in order to produce,

CHECKLIST

You can do many things to avoid excessive contamination of food and still maintain a varied, balanced diet that is conducive to good health.

✔ *Check food labels and avoid foods that have long lists of chemicals.*

✔ *Wash vegetables and fruits thoroughly to remove pesticide residues. (Special products are available for removing pesticides.)*

✔ *Choose organic produce and free-range chickens.*

✔ *Buy locally grown seasonal food whenever possible.*

✔ *Avoid unnecessary packaging and recycle as much packaging material as possible.*

✔ *Make your views known to your local produce markets to encourage them to stock organic produce.*

process, package, and transport many foodstuffs. This excessive consumption adds to the growing problem of global warming.

Only a small percentage of food is now locally grown and sold. Many fruits and vegetables are transported by air freight halfway around the world, and food grown in the United States may travel up and down or across the country many times before it eventually reaches the market. This reliance on transportation adds to air pollution and exacerbates climate changes, the long-term health effects of which could be devastating.

Ideally, we should all aim to buy as much locally grown fresh food as possible to reduce the amount of transportation required, concentrate on organic produce if possible, and limit the amount of processed and packaged foods we purchase.

FOOD STORAGE FOR HEALTH

Food is one of the main routes by which environmental contaminants and other toxic substances can enter the body and harm our general health. Some

packaging used for food may be harmful under certain circumstances. However, there are storage alternatives. Freezer paper or wax paper can be used for wrapping food, and parchment can be used instead of aluminum foil for baking. Food can be removed from plastic containers and packaging and stored in glass or ceramic jars and other containers.

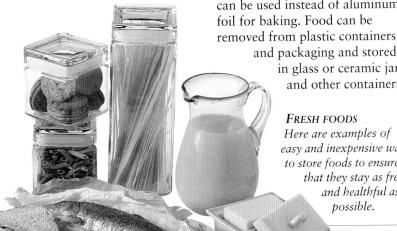

FRESH FOODS
Here are examples of easy and inexpensive ways to store foods to ensure that they stay as fresh and healthful as possible.

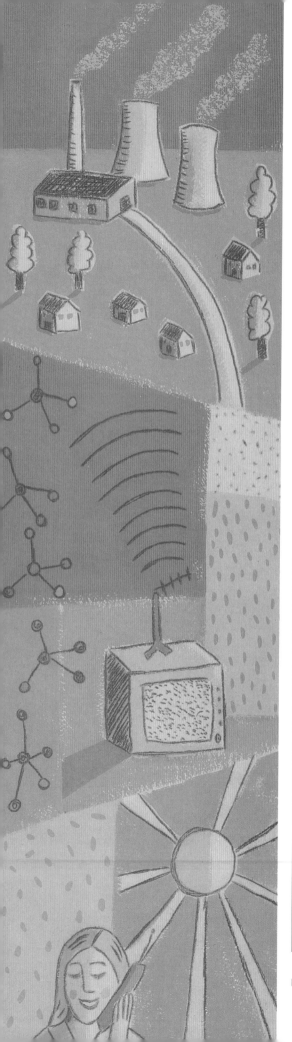

Radiation

We are constantly exposed to radiation from many sources, both natural—the sun, rocks, and soil—and man-made—domestic appliances, power lines, and medical equipment. Whether this exposure poses health risks is still highly controversial.

Radiation can be defined as the emission or transfer of energy in the form of light, heat, or electromagnetic waves. It includes electromagnetic radiation (EMR) and radioactivity. Many natural sources of radiation, such as the sun, are vital to life. But there are other forms found in the environment, both natural and man-made, that may pose a health risk. Scientists are investigating their possible long-term effects on health and seeking ways to minimize any potential dangers.

ELECTROMAGNETIC RADIATION

Electromagnetic radiation, the most widespread form of energy in nature, is also produced by man-made devices. The effects that natural forms of EMR have on health are well known, but there is growing concern about the possible impact of man-made sources of this energy.

EMR includes light, heat (also known as infrared radiation), X-rays, microwaves, and radio waves. The different forms of EMR can be distinguished by the lengths or

MICROWAVE OVENS

Microwave ovens cook and reheat food rapidly, which suits the busy lifestyle of many people today. They produce electromagnetic radiation, which can damage internal body organs. If you stay a safe distance from the oven, the risks from radiation are minimal.

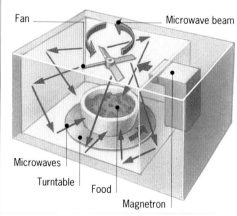

Fan — Microwave beam

Microwaves
Turntable | Food
Magnetron

HOW MICROWAVES WORK
A magnetron produces a beam of microwaves that strikes a spinning fan and reflects the waves into the food. The waves pass through the food container to heat the food only.

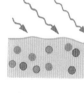

Microwaves penetrate water molecules in the food, so it cooks from the inside out.

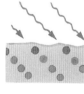

Microwaves cause the water molecules to align rapidly and then reverse alignment.

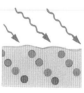

This quick and repeated vibration and twisting of the water molecules produces heat.

HOW A MOBILE (CELLULAR) PHONE WORKS

Mobile phones have built-in radio receivers and transmitters. A transmitter in the phone connects the call to a base station. From there the call is connected to a telephone network, and a local transmitter sends incoming signals to a radio receiver in the target phone. Some of the radio waves are absorbed by the phone user's head, and it is feared that these could cause damage to the brain.

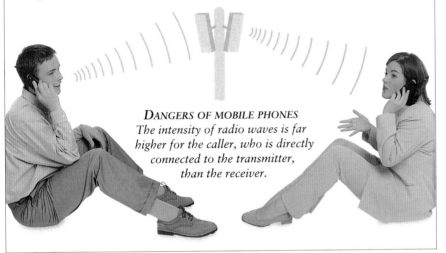

DANGERS OF MOBILE PHONES
The intensity of radio waves is far higher for the caller, who is directly connected to the transmitter, than the receiver.

frequencies of their waves. The whole range of electromagnetic radiation is known as the electro-magnetic spectrum. The most powerful natural source of EMR is the sun, which constantly bombards the earth with the entire spectrum of radiation. The sun produces many forms of radiation, but its ultraviolet rays, which cause suntan and sun-burn (see page 60), pose the greatest risk to health.

Sources of EMR

Many commonplace devices are powerful sources of invisible EMR. Microwave ovens generate short electromagnetic waves that are strong enough to cook food. They cause the water molecules in food to vibrate so fast that the friction generated causes the food to heat up. Microwaves mainly stay inside the oven, but if the oven door is damaged or faulty, they can leak out. These waves disperse quickly and are harmless at a distance, but at close range they can generate heat in the body that may damage internal

organs. They can also cause cataracts. As a general rule, it is advisable to stay at least an arm's length from a microwave oven while it is operat-ing. To avoid health risks, you can use a microwave detector regularly to check the safety of the oven.

Outdoors, radio waves are beamed nonstop from powerful towers and radar antennae. These are normally sited in remote locations, and any EMR that reaches the public is very weak. However, in recent years the increasing use of cellular phones has raised the prospect of a new hazard. Many people are concerned about the growing number of transmission towers, or base stations, erected close to homes, schools, and offices. But of even more concern is the effect of radio waves emitted from the handset itself.

In Australia there has been an increase in brain tumors over the past decade, the period when mobile phones became very popular; brain cancers have risen by 60 percent in women and 50 percent in men during this period. The British

government has launched a research program into the possible risks from mobile phones, which has yielded a great deal of information, especially about the way radio waves pass through the brain. Research is continuing worldwide, and both the World Health Organization and the European Community have substantial projects underway.

Some scientists maintain that radio waves do not have enough energy to break the strands of DNA in the nucleus of body cells, a possible starting point for cancer, but they may facilitate a cancer that has already formed. More research is needed, but in the meantime, people who have such phones should try to limit their use of them.

MEDICAL RADIATION

Several forms of radiation are employed in medicine. X-rays are the longest established and most widely used form. There are also gamma rays and other types of radioactive isotopes. Since their discovery in 1895, X-rays have been widely used not only in medicine but also in industry, scientific research, even art galleries to examine old paintings.

X-rays are useful in medical imaging because they pass through the tissues of the body but are stopped by the bones, which show

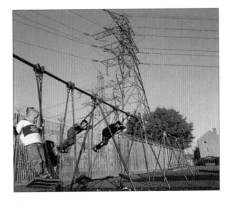

ELECTROMAGNETIC RADIATION
Transmitter poles for electricity emit electromagnetic radiation, and these emissions have generated a considerable amount of concern about their safety.

up on a photographic film. When the film is developed, it produces a picture of certain internal structures of the body.

X-rays and gamma rays can also be used to destroy cancerous growths. Early X-ray machines were fairly inaccurate and generated high radiation levels. Modern equipment is more sophisticated; it functions with minimum levels of radiation and is computer controlled, which ensures that the X-rays are targeted directly on the cancer, thus reducing the risk to neighboring tissues. Methods for reducing radiation further are still being researched. Studies by the medical professions have led to a reduction in average doses for most X-ray examinations by 30 percent since the mid-1980s.

Risks from radiation

Any radiation dose, however small, carries a risk of cancer, so it follows that X-rays could also be harmful.

For this reason X-rays are done only if there is a clear clinical need or justification. They must be carried out according to the best current practices and involve radiation doses that are as low as possible. This is called optimization. If these rules are followed, the benefits of X-rays greatly outweigh the risks.

Levels of radiation from X-rays can be compared with those from natural background radiation, to which everyone is constantly exposed. For example, low-dose X-rays, such as those of the teeth, are equivalent to the radiation levels received in a few days from natural sources. They produce an increased risk of cancer of about one in a million. Procedures involving higher doses or numerous X-rays and also computed tomography (CT) scans, in which multiple X-rays create a three-dimensional view of the body, involve doses equivalent to a few years of natural radiation. The cancer risk

then becomes one in a few thousand. The bottom line is always to approach the use of X-rays with some caution.

ELECTROMAGNETIC FIELDS

Electromagnetic fields (EMFs) differ from electromagnetic radiation. Although electricity and magnetism are closely related forces, a magnetic field generates electricity, and an electric current produces magnetism (or electromagnetism). Molecules within these fields, including those in living tissue, attempt to align themselves with the force lines.

Magnetism is a force that has existed in nature throughout time; the earth itself is a giant magnet, so living creatures have evolved with it. Man-made EMFs exist only while an electric current is on, and they are constantly changing or alternating direction. It is only within the past 100 years that these EMFs have played a part in human life.

The growing use of electrical equipment, both at home and in industry, has led to a huge increase in EMFs that are impossible to avoid. Power lines and household wiring produce EMFs, as do electrical appliances. The EMF acting on a person may increase by 25 times when an electric stove is switched on and by 1,000 times when that person walks under power lines.

Environmental scientists are concerned about the possible effects that a powerful and constantly changing electric field may have on human tissue. The World Health Organization launched its International EMF Project in May 1996 to assess the possible health risks from EMFs, with research scheduled to last for five years.

Although risks to health from EMFs have not been established, Swedish authorities recommend a cautious approach. They say that the design and siting of new facilities should be aimed at limiting exposure to reduce the risk of injury to human

---

MEDICAL X-RAYS

X-rays are frequently used in hospitals to take pictures of bones and organs in order to detect any damage or disease. Too much radiation can cause cancer.

However, the areas of the patient's body not being X-rayed are protected by thick lead screens, and the benefits of X-rays usually outweigh any minor risks.

TO MAKE AN X-RAY PICTURE X-rays pass through the body onto a photographic film placed behind the patient (right). Bones and dense tissue show up on the final photograph (below) because they absorb the X-rays.

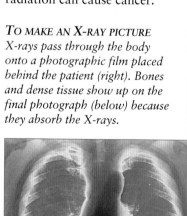

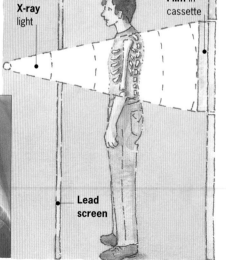

X-ray light

Film in cassette

Lead screen

NUCLEAR POWER

Hailed as an inexpensive and readily renewable alternative to fossil fuels when it was first developed, nuclear power has been shown to be extremely hazardous if mishandled, and the risks to health are long-lasting. The disaster at Chernobyl in Ukraine in 1986 focused worldwide attention on the dangers, but some groups have long campaigned for recognition of health risks they believe are associated with living near sources of nuclear power and waste. Despite fairly high safety standards in the West, some governments are now reviewing the future of their nuclear programs.

beings. When exposures from existing electrical facilities deviate significantly from what is normal, measures to reduce exposure should be taken when they can be carried out at reasonable cost.

For the individual, measures to reduce exposure to EMFs are limited. You can, in principle, avoid living near power plants and might object to new power lines being installed in your area. But if you want electricity in your home, there is little you can do to avoid EMFs.

Exposure to EMFs from domestic appliances varies. Washing machines, clothes dryers, and ovens perform their function while the user does something else. Vacuum cleaners and hair dryers are generally used for only a short time, while televisions and radios are used at a distance. Those who are concerned about EMFs from household appliances can try to limit their individual exposure, but as yet no national or international body has advocated these measures. Computers generate fairly powerful electromagnetic fields and can be tiring and stressful to use

over long periods. It makes sense, therefore, to take regular breaks away from the computer and also use a screen filter to protect yourself from the electromagnetic emissions.

A study of 3,000 children in Great Britain is currently looking for a link between cancer and various environmental factors, including EMFs, as well as lifestyle, radiation, chemicals, and viruses. Several causes of cancer in children have been suggested, including exposure to harmful radiation or chemicals during fetal development or soon after birth and exposure to infection or EMFs during early life.

RADIOACTIVE GAS

Natural radioactivity is all around us, usually at a harmless level. An exception is the naturally occurring radioactive gas known as radon. Released by the breakdown of uranium in rock, soil, and water, radon is the second leading cause of deaths from lung cancer annually in the United States. Outdoors, radon disperses rapidly, so levels remain low, but in enclosed spaces, such as buildings and mines, it can become dangerously concentrated. Nearly 1 in 15 homes in this country is believed to have elevated radon levels.

Radon is radioactive but chemically inert and does not normally form chemical compounds. It changes into solid radioactive particles that remain suspended in air. When inhaled, they irradiate the lung tissues with alpha particles. Radon also dissolves in water. Dangerous concentrations in municipal water supplies are very rare, but well water can pose a risk.

Widespread lung disease among silver miners in the Schneeberg region of Germany was noticed by Paracelsus in the 16th century. But radon itself was not discovered until 1900 by physicist Friedrich Dorn. High levels of radon were measured in the Schneeberg mines in 1901, and a theory was proposed that radon

was the cause. Later studies of radon in homes by the Swedish Radiation Protection Institute showed the public was also at risk.

Protecting yourself

The Environmental Protection Agency (EPA) has set the maximum acceptable standard for indoor radon at 4 picoCuries per liter (4pCi/L). The only way to ascertain the level present in a building is to test for it. The surgeon general recommends testing schools and all homes below the third floor. Inexpensive do-it-yourself kits are available from catalogs and at hardware stores, or you can have a professional do it.

There are two ways to test—short-term and long-term. Short-term tests remain in the home for 2 to 90 days; long-term tests remain for more than 90 days and are generally more accurate because radon levels can vary from day to day. The test kit is placed in a room that is used regularly on the lowest level of the home. For a short-term test, outside doors and windows should be kept closed as much as possible.

Measures to reduce radon concentrations include sealing cracks in floors and walls; installing a low-power fan to extract radon through a pipe; and in new houses, constructing an airtight membrane across the floor and through the walls. Consult a radon expert for the best approach.

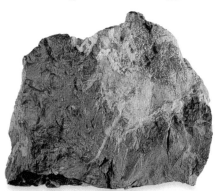

RADIOACTIVE ROCK
Radon is a radioactive gas released from the breakdown of uranium in rock, soil, and water; it can cause lung cancer.

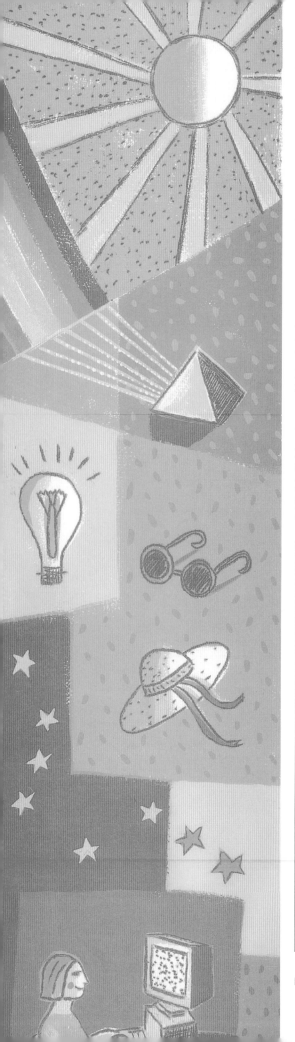

Light

Light—from both natural and man-made sources—is all around you, and it is easy to take it for granted. But its effects can be both beneficial and potentially harmful. Understanding the properties of light can help you to live with it safely.

Our most important source of light is the sun, which emits vast amounts of energy as heat and light. It provides the energy for plants to grow; plants in turn provide food (energy) for animals, including humans.

SIGHT

When a baby is born, the visual pathway is incomplete. In order for sight to develop properly, light must pass through the transparent structures of the eye to stimulate the brain cells. If anything obstructs this pathway, such as a bandage, it must be removed within the child's first year of life. Otherwise the brain cells normally dedicated to receiving light become devoted to other tasks, and the child may become permanently blind, even though the eyes themselves may be perfectly healthy.

Much of what we see results from light reflected from objects we are looking at. Lighter-colored objects reflect light and so seem brighter, while darker objects absorb light. Light-colored clothes are cooler to

---

ANATOMY OF THE EYE

Light rays enter the eye through the pupil and are focused by the lens and cornea to form an image on the retina. A series of nervous impulses is translated by the brain to produce a single image.

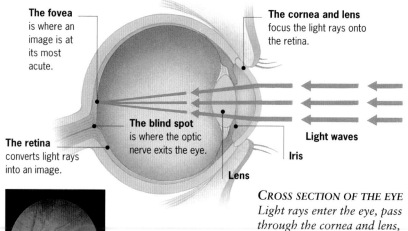

The fovea is where an image is at its most acute.

The cornea and lens focus the light rays onto the retina.

The retina converts light rays into an image.

The blind spot is where the optic nerve exits the eye.

Light waves

Iris

Lens

THE BLIND SPOT
At left is a microscopic image of the blind spot, the point where the optic nerve exits the eye.

CROSS SECTION OF THE EYE
Light rays enter the eye, pass through the cornea and lens, and converge at a point on the retina called the fovea, where the focused image is at its most acute. Damage to the fovea can cause blindness.

ULTRAVIOLET RADIATION

There are three principal wavelengths of ultraviolet light: UVA, UVB, and UVC. It is mostly the UVA rays that reach the ground and give us a suntan. UVB and UVC rays are potentially the most harmful because they have shorter waves, but they are usually blocked by ozone in the atmosphere. This is why a hole discovered in the ozone layer is of such concern; it means the earth is no longer fully protected from the most dangerous UV rays.

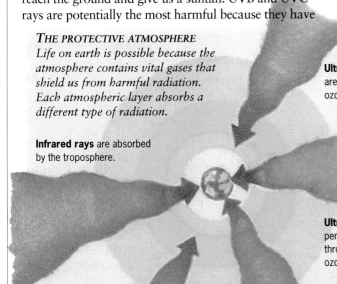

THE PROTECTIVE ATMOSPHERE
Life on earth is possible because the atmosphere contains vital gases that shield us from harmful radiation. Each atmospheric layer absorbs a different type of radiation.

Infrared rays are absorbed by the troposphere.

Ultraviolet rays are absorbed by the ozone layer.

Ultraviolet rays penetrate the earth through holes in the ozone layer.

Radio shortwaves and light waves reach the earth.

The thermo-sphere traps radio long waves.

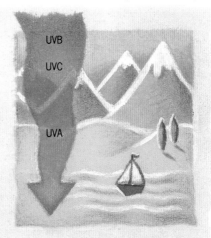

HARMFUL ULTRAVIOLET RAYS
The sun's rays are at their most intense at high elevations, where the thinner atmosphere provides little protection from them.

wear because they reflect the sun's infrared (heat) rays, whereas dark clothes tend to absorb them.

The cornea and the crystalline lens focus light on a light-sensitive layer of the eye called the retina to produce an upside-down image. Light waves converge at the fovea, and cells inside the retina called rods and cones respond to the light by sending nerve impulses along the optic nerve to the brain. It is in the brain where they are interpreted into readable images. The retina contains about 120 million rods and 7 million cones. The rods work best in dim light and are responsive to move-ment, whereas the cones are responsible for color vision and enable you to see detail.

Muscles in the iris control the amount of light entering the eye and alter the size of the pupil, which lets in light. In dim light the pupil gets larger; in bright light it gets smaller.

THE HEALTHY EFFECTS OF SUNLIGHT

Ultraviolet (UV) rays from the sun produce vitamin D in the skin, which is vital for the healthy development and maintenance of bones and teeth in both children and adults.

In urban areas much of the therapeutic effect of the sun's rays is filtered out by moisture, dust, and smoke in the air. This can have a harmful effect during childhood, particularly among youngsters who have inadequate diets. Disabling diseases such as rickets are traceable in part to lack of sunlight. Night-shift workers are particularly at risk from a similar disorder called osteomalacia, which affects adults.

To prevent bone disorders, it is essential that everyone, but especially young children, obtain sunshine on a regular basis. Much of the benefit of sunshine is derived from its UV rays,

but natural sunshine is preferable to the rays produced by a UV lamp, which can be too intense and may increase the risk of skin cancer. In northern latitudes, where winters can bring up to 24 hours of darkness, it is often necessary to expose children

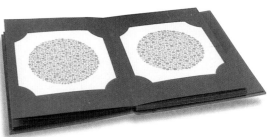

COLOR BLINDNESS
Color blindness, an inability to distinguish between red and green, affects 1 in 15 boys and 1 in 100 girls. The Ishihara test plate, shown above, is used to detect color blindness. People who have normal vision are able to distinguish the numbers in orange and red dots among the green and blue dots.

to UV lamps on a regular basis to provide them with an adequate source of vitamin D.

The beneficial effects of light are used in various medical treatments. Light therapy is used to relieve a depressive condition called seasonal affective disorder (SAD), which is associated with lack of sunlight. UV light and sunlight are also employed in the treatment of skin disorders, such as vitiligo and psoriasis. And visible blue light is used to treat jaundice in newborn babies.

THE UNHEALTHY EFFECTS OF SUNLIGHT

Extreme heat from the sun can cause disorders like heat exhaustion and sunstroke. Heat exhaustion is most likely to occur in people who are working or playing sports during hot weather and can be made worse by an inadequate intake of water and salt, which are lost through sweat. A humid atmosphere, which interferes with the body's natural cooling systems, increases the likelihood of becoming overheated. Heat exhaustion causes fatigue, nausea,

headache, and sometimes fainting. It is best treated by letting the sufferer rest in a cool, darkened room. A wet compress on the head will help the person cool down; giving a weak saltwater solution (¼ teaspoon salt in 2 cups water) to sip will restore the electrolyte balance.

Sunstroke is a far more serious condition because the body becomes dangerously overheated. A sufferer should be sponged with cold water or wrapped in a wet sheet to bring the body temperature down and given emergency medical aid.

Excessive exposure to UV rays can cause sunburn. Special cells in the skin called melanocytes produce a pigment called melanin, which helps to protect the skin against UV light. Darker-skinned people produce more melanin and thus have more natural protection from the sun than individuals with paler complexions.

UV rays can also lead to skin cancer, particularly among persons who are lighter skinned, who work outdoors, or have sun-induced skin damage. Sunburn, especially in childhood, increases this risk, so

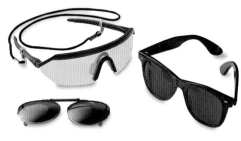

EYE PROTECTION
Eyes must be protected from ultraviolet light by wearing sunglasses or contact lenses that have been coated with a good-quality UV block.

children must always be fully protected from the sun with a hat and sun cream. There are various forms of skin cancer, but the most dangerous type is malignant melanoma, which starts in the melanocytes. Skin tumors can be removed with minor surgery, a laser, or freezing, or can be treated with anticancer drugs applied to the skin.

Lifelong sun protection is the key to prevention. In bright sunlight, especially in the summer, wear a broad-brimmed hat and apply a suitable sunblock to all exposed skin. The amount of protection given by a sunblock is indicated by its sun protection factor (SPF). Very fair-skinned people should use a sunblock with at least a factor of 15 and keep out of direct sunlight whenever possible. Everyone should avoid sunbathing between 10:00 A.M. and 3.00 P.M., which is the period when the sun is at its most intense. Visits to tanning salons and other exposure to intense artificial UV light should also be limited.

THE EFFECTS OF SUNLIGHT ON YOUR EYES

UV radiation can damage eyes. A painful condition called actinic keratopathy, or snow blindness, is caused by bright light reflected from light surfaces—for example, snow, ice, or sand. UV rays burn the cornea and conjunctiva, the membrane that covers the surface of the eye, and cause temporary blindness. The

COMPARING LIGHT SYSTEMS

By using the spectral distribution of the colors of daylight, you can see how different artificial lights compare. Full-spectrum lamps offer the closest light to daylight, while in comparison, fluorescent tubes tend to create a different, "cold" light, consisting of quite a bit more yellow, less blue, and much less red.

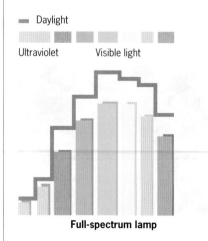

Daylight

Ultraviolet   Visible light

Full-spectrum lamp

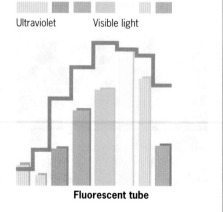

Ultraviolet   Visible light

Fluorescent tube

damage can occur when arc welding, glassblowing, skiing, or using tanning beds. Protective goggles should always be worn with these activities. UV radiation can also cause cataracts—cloudy areas in the crystalline lens of the eye that result in reduced vision and eventually blindness. A pterygium—a fold of tissue on the conjunctiva that affects the visual center—is also caused by UV radiation. Surgery can usually correct both problems.

Burn damage to the fovea, the most sensitive point on the retina, can result from looking at an eclipse of the sun with the naked eye. The damage is permanent and causes impaired visual activity, which may include a permanent black spot in the center of the field of vision. The lens of the eye can absorb some harmful rays, but a cataract could still develop. Never look directly at an eclipse or its reflection, even through smoked glass.

LIGHT POLLUTION

The stars are just as bright now as they ever were, but in many parts of the world, especially urban areas, they no longer seem so. Much of the night sky is now hidden behind a light haze caused by street lights and artificial light sources reflecting off the atmosphere. Called light pollution, this is of special concern to astronomers, who must move to increasingly remote locations to escape its effect. But the public loses out as well by missing the beauty of the night sky. Astronomers believe that much of this light pollution is unnecessary and could be minimized by designing artificial light fixtures to reflect downward, where the light is needed, not upward toward space.

EYE CARE WHEN USING COMPUTERS

There is little evidence, even after extensive research, that computer screens, also called monitors or visual display units (VDUs), cause eye disease or permanent damage to the eyes. But the fatigue brought on by intensive computer work can result in eye discomfort. Because the monitor gives your eyes demanding tasks, it may also make you aware of an eye problem you had not noticed before. This condition is made worse if the screen is badly positioned or the workplace is poorly lit. For this reason it is advisable to have an annual eye examination if you work at a computer terminal for long periods of time.

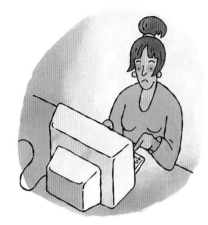

BOGGLE-EYED
Long periods of computer work can exacerbate eye problems and cause eye fatigue symptoms, such as double vision. Regular breaks are essential.

ARTIFICIAL LIGHT
Light is produced artificially with electricity or fire. The production of light by a hot object, such as a bulb's filament, a candle's flame, or the sun's surface, is called incandescence. Luminescence is the collective name for other ways of producing light. Fireflies, for instance, produce chemicals that react to create light called bioluminescence. Fluorescence occurs when substances absorb light briefly, then release it. Some detergents contain fluorescent chemicals that make clothes look brighter.

Electric lights
An incandescent lightbulb is made of a thin coil of special resistance wire containing the metal tungsten, which can withstand very high temperatures. The wire glows at more than 2,500°C (4,530°F) when electricity flows along it. A special gas mixture inside the glass or a vacuum prevents the wire from burning out too quickly.

A fluorescent bulb produces more light from a given amount of electricity than an incandescent bulb. The tube is filled with a vapor of mercury. The metal electrode gives off a beam of invisible, electrically charged particles called electrons. When an electron hits a mercury atom, it momentarily knocks one of the mercury electrons out of position. This creates a burst of UV light, which is turned into visible light by the tube's internal coating. The light in a neon tube is produced by electroluminescence. When passed through the neon, electrical energy causes the gas atoms to emit light.

Laser
A laser—light amplification by stimulated emission of radiation—is an intense beam of light. High-voltage electricity passes through a glass tube containing a mixture of gases, such as helium and neon. The electricity stimulates the gas atoms to give off tiny packets of light called photons. These stimulate other atoms to emit photons. Mirrors reflect most of the light back into the gas for further amplification. A partially silvered mirror at one end permits escape of a narrow beam of intensely bright, pure, single-color light called a laser beam.

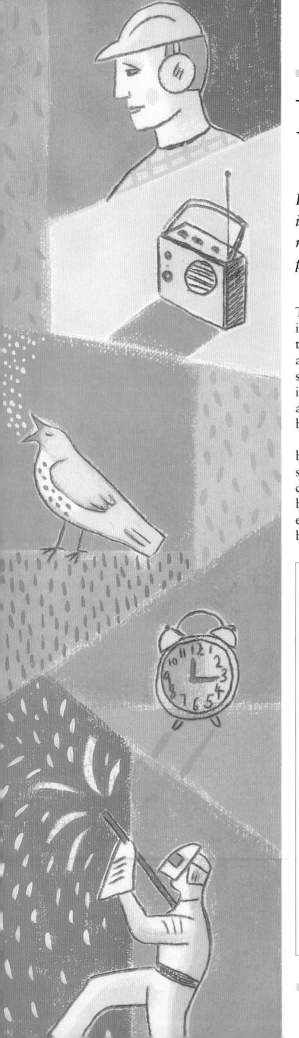

Noise

Persistently loud, jarring, or intrusive noise is a growing menace in society and a common cause of irritation, disturbed sleep, and neighborhood disputes. Tackling chronic noise nuisance takes planning, diplomacy, and consideration on all sides.

The sounds of human activities, including construction work, road traffic, leisure pursuits on watercraft and snowmobiles, outdoor events such as concerts, and—perhaps most intrusive—noise from neighbors, appear to be growing steadily in both volume and irritation factor.

Moderate amounts of noise can be tolerable, even beneficial and stimulating; for example, a car radio can relieve tedium on a long and boring journey. And some noise is essential. How many people would be late for work without alarm clocks? But unwanted sounds, particularly when they are loud, can be distracting, annoying, and if excessive, harmful to well-being. These types of sounds seem to be increasing. In England and Wales, for instance, complaints made to local authorities about noisy neighbors climbed from 55,000 in 1985 to more than 164,000 in 1995.

Annoyance is the most common reaction to noise. Whether or not a sound is annoying depends on many factors—the time that it occurs, its character, its duration,

---

ANATOMY OF THE EAR

The ear has three parts: the outer ear, which is visible and protective and funnels sound; the middle ear, which sends vibrations to the inner ear; and the inner ear, which transmits messages to the brain.

EAR STRUCTURE
When sound waves enter the ear, the eardrum vibrates. Three small bones transmit these vibrations to the inner ear, from which nerve messages are sent to the brain to create sound.

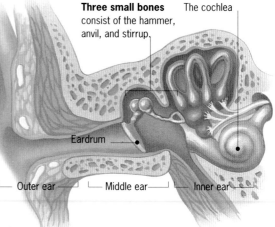

Three small bones consist of the hammer, anvil, and stirrup.

The cochlea

Eardrum

Outer ear — Middle ear — Inner ear

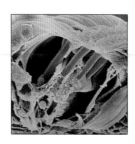

HAIR CELLS
The cochlea contains the spiral organ of Corti, the organ of hearing. Four rows of hair cells in the Corti translate the vibrations into nerve impulses.

NOISE POLLUTION

Many of the sounds that surround us every day are pleasant and essential to a healthy lifestyle, but when sound becomes noise, it can be very stressful. Thanks to technology, life is noisier than ever before. There are more vehicles on the road and more airplanes in the sky, and people are using gadgets and pleasure vehicles to create more noise. It can often be impossible to find a peaceful space. Noise pollution is now seen as a real health hazard, and it is being taken very seriously in many communities.

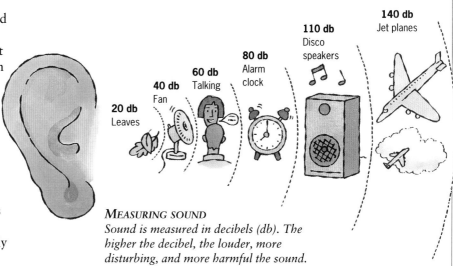

20 db Leaves
40 db Fan
60 db Talking
80 db Alarm clock
110 db Disco speakers
140 db Jet planes

MEASURING SOUND
Sound is measured in decibels (db). The higher the decibel, the louder, more disturbing, and more harmful the sound.

how repetitive it is, and not the least, whether or not it can be controlled. Uncontrollable noise, especially in the home, is often seen as an invasion of privacy. If a noise regularly interferes with sleep, it can cause stress and lower the immune system enough to result in illness.

HOW SOUND IS MADE

Sound is a succession of airwaves—alternating areas of compression (high pressure) and rarifaction (low pressure)—that spread out from a source such as a loudspeaker, just like the peaks and troughs of the ripples on a pond. Noise meters have sensitive microphones to measure these pressure differences. The unit of measurement is the decibel (db). Complete silence, when there is no audible pressure fluctuation, is represented by 0 db; a soft whisper measures 30 db; normal conversation measures about 60 db; a noisy restaurant may measure 80 db, and a car horn nearby, 120 db. Higher up the scale near the threshold of pain is a gunshot in close proximity, which comes in at 140 db.

Sound frequency is the speed with which airwaves oscillate, or vibrate. The more rapidly that high pressure is exchanged for low pressure, the higher the frequency and the higher the pitch of the sound. Most people can hear sounds that range from 20 Hertz (Hz), or cycles per second, to 20,000 Hz, although this range lessens with age.

Loudness is the main factor in defining how intrusive a sound is. An increase in sound pressure of 10 db equates to a doubling of loudness. But how loudly a sound is perceived will also depend on its frequency; a high-pitched sound seems much louder than a low-pitched one.

EFFECTS OF NOISE ON HEARING

While loudness is the major cause of annoyance, it is sound pressure—the amount of energy in sound—that can cause damage. The most serious danger from noise is deafness, which may be irreversible. This is known as presbycusis and is distinct from the normal deterioration of hearing that results from aging. Noise-induced hearing losses can be either temporary or permanent.

Temporary hearing loss

A short-term loss of hearing may be experienced by someone who has been exposed to loud noise for a relatively short period, such as at a rock concert. Sound pressures of 90 db or more experienced for a few minutes are usually enough to cause an effect called noise-induced temporary threshold shift, or NITTS. This may last for about half an hour after the noise stops. Fortunately, normal hearing usually returns.

Permanent hearing loss

Sudden traumatic deafness can be caused by being in close proximity to an explosion. But in less dramatic cases, the relationship between repeated bouts of temporary hearing loss and permanent damage is uncertain. It is clear, however, that

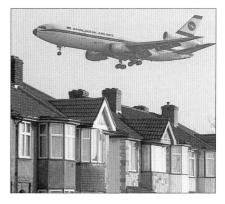

LIFE UNDER THE FLIGHT PATH
Living near an airport or under a flight path can be very disturbing. The noise not only is intrusive but also can disrupt everyday life and a peaceful night's sleep.

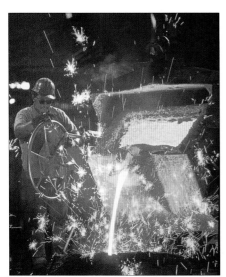

NOISE IN THE WORKPLACE
The risks of excessive noise are often overlooked in the workplace. This steelworker is wearing heat-resistant gloves and head and eye protection, yet his ears are exposed to dangerous noise levels.

more prolonged or repeated exposure to loud noise can result in an irreversible shift in the threshold of hearing. This is called noise-induced permanent threshold shift, or NIPTS, and is caused by damage to the Corti—fine hair cells—of the inner ear. It is estimated that one in five teenagers today already suffers from some hearing loss.

Individual susceptibility varies, so it is impossible to predict accurately what level of exposure to noise will be damaging. It usually takes a few years to become apparent and first tends to affect only the ability to hear higher-frequency sounds.

While prolonged workplace exposure to noise levels above 60 db may be annoying, risk of permanent damage if it remains below 75 db over an eight-hour period is thought to be negligible. Above this level workers must take appropriate precautions, such as wearing ear protectors. However, some employees, such as disc jockeys, bartenders, and waitresses, may find it difficult to take appropriate safety steps in their line of work.

Many states have passed antinoise laws or have delegated this power to local governments, and there are thousands of regulations now in effect. Most of them specify decibel limits on amplified speech or music and contain general provisions against both loud and annoying sounds.

OTHER EFFECTS OF NOISE ON HEALTH

In addition to causing hearing loss, noise can be damaging to health in a number of ways. These include effects on sleep, concentration, and the heart. But some of these effects are hard to establish with certainty.

Effects of noise on sleep

One harmful result of noise, with which everyone is familiar, occurs when it delays or prevents sleep or causes a sleeper to waken. Noise can also cause changes in the rhythm of sleep, leading to restlessness and resulting in fatigue and impaired performance, particularly of routine tasks, the following day.

Depending on its degree, disturbed sleep can also lead to mood swings and depression during the day. Individual susceptibility varies, and there is evidence that some people grow less vulnerable to waking over time. However, the elderly, who are often light sleepers, may be more prone to disturbance. The problem seems to be related more to the number of noisy events during the night than to the loudness of the sound. Women seem to suffer sleep disturbances more than men, while children appear to be least affected.

Sleep deprivation from noise does affect well-being and quality of life, but the evidence that it causes serious physical health problems is less clear-cut. However, research into the sleep patterns of people who are disturbed by shift work, air travel, or sleep disorders suggests there may be a range of ill effects. These include reduced ability to concentrate, leading to an increased risk of

accidents, and a higher incidence of stress-related disorders, such as heart disease and elevated blood pressure.

Background noise

Some background noises are meant to be distracting; an example is music played in factories for production-line workers. In other circumstances background noise can be stimulating, if only subliminally, that is, at an unconscious level. The music played in stores falls into this category. But certain background noises, even at low levels, can make it harder to concentrate on the task at hand and can impair performance, principally by being distracting. This is particularly true of speech. Complicated tasks are the most affected, especially multifaceted ones that require planning.

Noise also hinders communication, by making it harder to hear others talking and vice versa. Studies of schoolchildren living near airports suggest negative effects on learning skills and long-term memory.

Cardiovascular effects

More worrisome, perhaps, are the physiological reactions to noise, which may include elevated heart rate and blood pressure. These reactions most often occur in

---

NOISIEST OCCUPATIONS

According to the U.S. National Institute of Occupational Health and Safety (NIOHS), the noisiest jobs are in the logging and lumber industries, textile production, the petroleum and coal industries, food and food-related industries, and furniture manufacturing. The NIOHS estimates that 14 percent of the U.S. workforce is employed in places where noise levels commonly exceed the level at which impairment can occur.

Some drugs, including many antibiotics, are ototoxic and can indirectly lead to deafness because they lower the sound threshold at which hearing damage can occur.

response to sudden loud noises as part of the body's "fight or flight" stress response, which causes the body to produce an excess of adrenal hormones. The elevation in hormones can in turn lead to other responses, such as an increase in heart and breathing rates. The same reaction to sudden noise has been observed in people during sleep, but in both cases normal levels usually return when the stimulus is removed.

Elevated blood pressure has also been observed in workers who are exposed to loud noise over long periods of time. However, it is not clear to what extent this is a result of the noise itself or other stressful workplace or external factors. Likewise, there is little evidence at

the present time to prove that environmental noise can lead to higher blood pressure.

Mental health

We've all heard the complaint "That noise is driving me crazy," but the evidence linking noise and mental illness is actually very slim. While noise can certainly induce stress, there is no evidence to suggest that it leads directly to mental illness. There is some evidence, however, that noise-sensitive people are more prone to mental illness and that the effects of noise may be more pronounced in some mentally ill persons.

NOISE CONTROL

There are various methods of noise control, but the ideal one is to reduce the noise emissions at their source.

The conditions that are set on plans for potentially noisy developments often stipulate noise limits to be observed along their boundaries. Similar limits imposed on the noise from car engines now mean that more noise is generated by the

contact of tires with the road at urban speeds. (Hope is in the offing; the Japanese are developing a quieter tire that has shock-absorbing rubber between the rim and the disc.)

Sometimes noisy processes can be replaced by quieter ones. If it is not possible to reduce a noise at its source, screening it may reduce its effects. The insulating jackets now fitted to road drills are a good example of this technique, as are the sound barrier walls that now line many highways, shielding nearby houses from the traffic roar. A line of trees with dense foliage, such as conifers, planted between your house and the road can also muffle traffic noise (see page 89).

Other attempts can be made to separate the sources of noise from the people who are most likely to be affected by it. For example, a common aim of land-use planning is to avoid conflicting uses of neighboring parcels of land. One way is to create separate zones for industrial and residential uses. But this is inevitably a long-term process.

WHEN YOU SHOULD WEAR EAR PROTECTION

Prolonged exposure to loud noise can cause a variety of health problems, from temporary and permanent hearing loss to stress. People who are surrounded constantly by noise at home or work should wear ear protection to prevent any long-term damage. Below are examples of situations that demand ear protection.

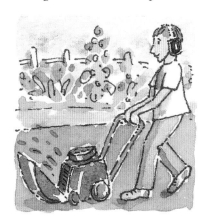

LAWN MOWING
Lawn mowers are fairly noisy, so it is advisable to wear ear protection if you are mowing for long periods of time.

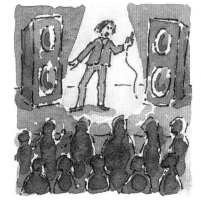

AT A CONCERT
Avoid standing too near the loud-speakers; the excessive noise can cause eventual hearing loss.

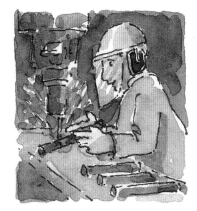

IN INDUSTRY
In a noisy working environment, it is essential to wear ear protection because of the constant loud noise.

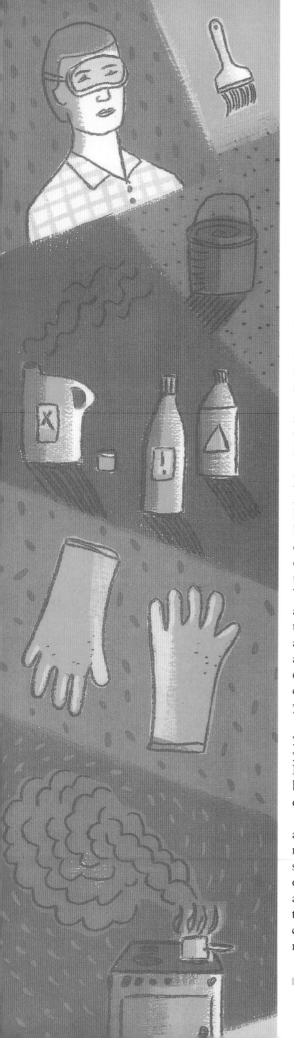

Hazards at home

You probably feel safest in the security of your own home, yet many chemicals found there are potentially dangerous. By knowing the risks, you can take more care when using household chemicals or, better still, avoid them altogether.

Many familiar household products and building materials that have been around for years are now known to be harmful. And new ones, including cleaning agents, pesticides, and do-it-yourself products, are being developed all the time. Some are being used excessively, even though little is known about their long-term effects on the environment.

Household cleaners

Many household products, including bleach, disinfectants, oven and toilet-bowl cleaners, drain decloggers, detergents, and glass cleaner, not only are toxic but can be lethal if not used in accordance with instructions. When using household cleaners, always follow the instructions, store them in a properly labeled container, and use them in well-ventilated areas. Oven cleaners can be especially harmful because they contain a highly corrosive ingredient; you must wear protective gloves.

If you spill a toxic substance on your skin, wash it off immediately. If you swallow any, seek medical help. Never mix anything with bleach because chlorine gas may be given off, and this can irritate the lungs.

Many stores and catalogs offer safe and ecologically friendly products, most of them made with natural substances, that can be used instead of toxic ones. These include nontoxic and chemical-free stain removers and toilet-bowl cleaners, biodegradable cleaning and polishing agents, and nontoxic odor absorbers.

Home pest control

In many cases home pesticides are unnecessary, and a nonchemical treatment would be better. For example, a common pesticide used in the home is a wood preservative that protects against rot—the underlying cause of which is dampness. Until the cause is tackled, chemical treatment may be advised but is not necessarily the best approach.

A group of compounds known as pyrethroids are less toxic than older chemicals but are still not necessarily safe. One pyrethroid, permethrin, can cause rash and a peripheral nervous system condition called paresthesia. Even pyrethrin, a natural form made from chrysanthemum flowers, can cause headaches, kidney problems, and fatigue and can trigger asthma in susceptible individuals.

For controlling pests in the garden, household-tip and gardening books offer formulas made with nontoxic ingredients that are found in most households—pepper and garlic, for example—and that won't harm the environment. There are also gadgets that emit repellent electronic sounds instead of dispensing poison.

The method of applying pesticides makes a difference. Flypaper, paste, dusting, and baited traps in the vicinity of nests are preferable to spraying. If spraying is unavoidable, water-based formulations are better than solvent-based ones. Official advice is that it is safe to re-enter the premises 48 hours after spraying, but some pesticides linger much longer.

IDENTIFYING HAZARDS IN THE HOME

Many dangers lie within the walls of a home in the form of cleaning agents, finishes on furniture, and paints. However, by taking a few simple precautions, you can ensure that your home is free from toxic substances. Good ventilation is essential to allow fresh air to circulate, and eco-friendly cleaning fluids reduce the amount of chemical fumes in the home. Gas appliances should be checked regularly.

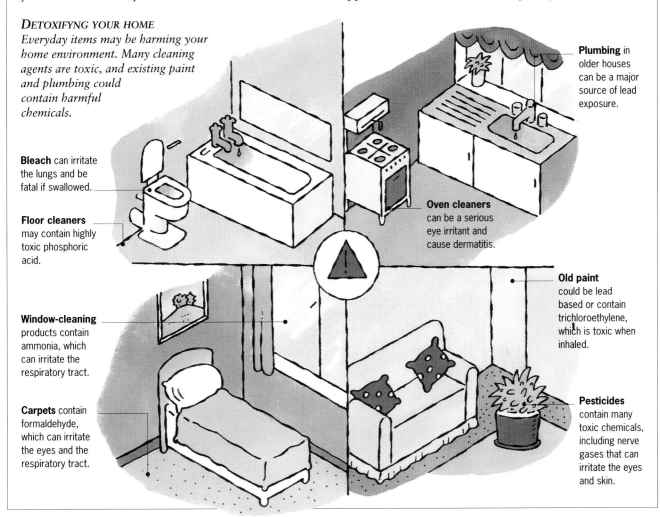

DETOXIFYNG YOUR HOME
Everyday items may be harming your home environment. Many cleaning agents are toxic, and existing paint and plumbing could contain harmful chemicals.

Plumbing in older houses can be a major source of lead exposure.

Bleach can irritate the lungs and be fatal if swallowed.

Floor cleaners may contain highly toxic phosphoric acid.

Oven cleaners can be a serious eye irritant and cause dermatitis.

Window-cleaning products contain ammonia, which can irritate the respiratory tract.

Old paint could be lead based or contain trichloroethylene, which is toxic when inhaled.

Carpets contain formaldehyde, which can irritate the eyes and the respiratory tract.

Pesticides contain many toxic chemicals, including nerve gases that can irritate the eyes and skin.

Other nontoxic approaches to dealing with household pests include filling in all the cracks around pipes and baseboards where they can enter and sprinkling boric acid around the base of kitchen cabinets to deter cockroaches . Also a cat can help control rodents in both the garden and home.

Dust
Dust, which has various harmful effects, can come from wood, cloth, cement, skin, flour, and tobacco and contain dust mites, fungal spores, pollen, animal dander, and insect particles. A cocktail of these materials and other chemicals can build up, especially in a sealed, centrally air-conditioned home. Symptoms of exposure include breathlessness, wheezing, sneezing, watery eyes, lethargy, headaches, stomach problems, and skin rash. The problem can be minimized by regular ventilation and cleaning.

Carbon monoxide
Gas heating and cooking appliances can give off carbon monoxide (CO), nitrogen oxides, and other toxic gases if they are improperly used, badly maintained, or faulty. Carbon monoxide, a colorless, odorless gas emitted when fossil fuel is burned inefficiently, can be lethal in a building that is inadequately ventilated. Low-level exposure can cause headaches, fatigue, and nausea. If you are suffering from these symptoms and have a gas appliance, see your doctor for a blood test and have the appliance checked. At higher exposures the onset of coma and death can be rapid and is hastened by exertion. Pregnant women, the

young, and the elderly are especially vulnerable. Victims should be removed from the area into fresh air and given medical attention.

Make sure there is good ventilation in any room that contains a gas appliance. If you suspect that the appliance is malfunctioning, switch it off until it has been inspected and repaired by a professional.

Lead-free paint

Modern lead-free paints are much safer than older ones that contain lead but still have potential hazards. Most of these arise when paint is applied or stored improperly. Once paint has dried completely, it is safe. But it is some time after application before it stops giving off fumes.

Excessive exposure to solvent-based paints can cause skin and respiratory symptoms, headaches, nausea, and other central nervous system problems. Studies of

professional painters suggest that there is also an increased risk of cancer. An area being painted should be well ventilated, with as many doors and windows as possible kept open. Do not eat while painting and, above all, never smoke; solvent-based paints are highly flammable. It is better if possible to use water-based paints because they are safer.

Formaldehyde

Formaldehyde is a colorless gas with a pungent odor that is used in building materials, such as particleboard, fiberboard, wall-insulation foam, and the preserving and disinfectant fluid formalin. It is also found in ink, adhesives, paint, and wallpaper and is often part of the finish on carpeting and fabrics.

Formaldehyde is a powerful respiratory irritant that causes coughing and shortness of breath. Effects can be felt by some people at

PROBLEMS WITH LEAD

Lead is a very toxic material when swallowed or inhaled. Symptoms of lead poisoning include fatigue, irritability, depression, sleep problems, stomach pains, constipation, persistent headaches, double vision, loss of appetite, and joint, muscle, and bone pain. Lead also affects reproductive health and, most seriously, very low levels of exposure can affect mental development in children. It is best to take precautions and have any traces of lead in the home removed by professionals.

exposures of only 0.5 parts per million, which is well below the officially permitted levels in most developed countries. At higher levels the gas can cause severe eye irritation, with blurred vision and watering, as well as skin problems, such as allergic dermatitis.

There has been a long-running controversy about the risk of cancer from formaldehyde. Evidence is accumulating that it can cause cancer of the nose at high exposure levels.

There has also been concern over possible dangers from medium-density fiberboard (MDF). This popular material consists of layers of wood fiber held together by resin. Formaldehyde is used in making the resin, and some excess may still exist in the finished product. This can be given off, or outgassed, over time or when the material is cut or shaped.

It is important to take precautions when using MDF. It should be bought from a reliable supplier who allows it to stand after manufacture until it is completely outgassed. Because very fine dust is given off when MDF is cut and shaped, carpenters should wear dust protection and work in a well-ventilated area, ideally in the open air. Once sealed with paint or varnish, MDF is perfectly safe.

ASBESTOS

Asbestos is a naturally occurring fire-resistant mineral used in about 3,000 home products, such as insulation for buildings and appliances, textured paint, carpet underlays, and roofing materials. It is generally safe when combined with other materials by means of a strong bonding agent but is dangerous if its fibers become loose and airborne. Some uses of asbestos have been banned; these include certain pipe coverings and patching compounds and materials for home construction.

If asbestos fibers are inhaled into the lungs, they may lodge and persist there for many years and eventually cause disease. It used to be thought that only miners and workers in heavy industry were at risk from asbestos diseases, but research shows that people exposed to asbestos in their homes

or schools may be in danger to some extent. Older properties should be surveyed for asbestos-containing building material; if any is found, it should be removed or sealed with professional help, depending on the type of asbestos and its condition.

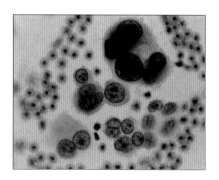

LUNG DISEASE
Inhalation of airborne asbestos can cause lung cancer and asbestosis, a scarring of the lungs that leads to breathing problems and heart failure.

CHAPTER 3

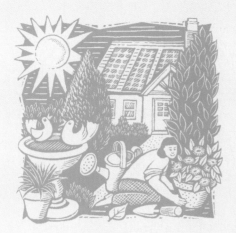

CHOOSING WHERE TO LIVE

In these days of smoke-free buildings in the city and agribusiness in the country, living in a rural area no longer has a cut-and-dried claim to being healthier than living in town. How healthy an environment is for you can depend as much on how well it suits your lifestyle and fulfills your needs as on more general factors, such as air quality. This chapter looks at some advantages and disadvantages of urban and rural living and highlights points to consider when choosing where you want to live.

URBAN VERSUS RURAL LIVING

Your community's environment can have a profound effect on your life and health. Choosing whether to live in the city, suburbs, or country may have major implications for your lifestyle.

Feeling comfortable in and connected to the environment in which you live is important for both your physical and emotional health. Whether you live in a city, the suburbs, or the country may be dictated by your employment. However, advances in computer technology and communications, such as e-mail and the Internet, have made the home office a more viable option and have also made it possible for many people to consider lifestyle options that would have been impossible in years past.

Some individuals who are dissatisfied with urban life may imagine that living in the country or suburbs will offer a less stressful and healthier environment, but there are many factors to be considered before making such a major change.

URBAN LIVING

Those who live in cities can enjoy many benefits and conveniences that are not readily available in the country or suburbs. For one, there is a greater variety of goods and services, and they are often less expensive and located within walking distance of

home. Some stores even offer delivery service because the population density makes it worthwhile. This factor could be important for you if you are elderly or infirm.

There are also more public support networks in urban areas because of the greater population. Examples are Meals on Wheels for the elderly or disabled, play groups and baby gyms for young children, and after-school and holiday activities for older children. Although such facilities do exist in some rural and suburban areas, they are usually on a much smaller scale, and choosing to use them may involve greater expense and time traveling a long distance.

Not only are stores and amenities diverse and convenient in cities, but cultural life is richer and more varied as well. Art shows, plays, live music, movies, and other forms of entertainment are more numerous, and museums are often of world-class stature. In addition, large cities tend to attract immigrants from many countries, providing a great diversity of cultures and cuisines.

Although a great exodus to the suburbs during the latter half of the last century left whole sections of cities abandoned or run

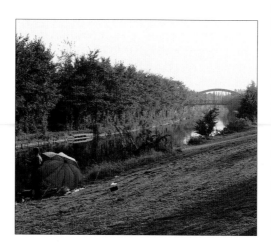

URBAN RENEWAL
In recent years many cities and large towns have shown imagination and initiative in developing new areas of green space. This parkland was a former London refuse dump and car-demolition site that was reclaimed for public use in 1981.

CREATIVE TRANSPORTATION SOLUTIONS

A number of local governments and enterprising entrepreneurs have developed creative strategies for reducing automobile usage and improving air quality in urban areas. In the German city of Bremen, for example, developers of a new housing enclave provided groups of households with a car to share on a rental basis. This significantly reduced the number of automobiles in the area and allowed the developers to build extra dwellings where they would otherwise have had to supply parking space. Because most of the householders require a car only for occasional shopping trips, the car-sharing system has worked well and saved them money. Other cities are now using vehicles with low emissions, such as electric buses.

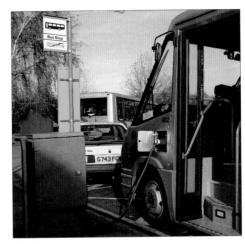

ON THE BUSES
This electrically powered bus in Oxford, England, produces no harmful emissions. It merely needs to be recharged after each run.

down, many of these areas have been rejuvenated, and they now provide a vibrant and inviting environment that has drawn many people back to city life.

Some cities also offer good access to nature. In recent years local governments have recognized the great importance of developing and maintaining woodlands and green open spaces for the public (and these spaces don't require any gardening chores on the part of the users). Many parks cater to the different needs of their users and have allocated separate areas in which young children can play safely, dog owners can let their dogs romp freely, and athletes can play football, tennis, and other games or go jogging around a circuit. In addition, quiet areas are usually set aside for people who want to read or simply sit in peace.

City dwellers enjoy the benefit of a strong infrastructure of public transportation as well. Urban areas usually have more frequent bus and train service, and in major cities there is often an underground metro system to make transportation as fast and convenient as possible.

Challenges of the city
There are some obvious disadvantages to city life. Large numbers of people going to and leaving work at roughly the same time create the commuter rush hour, which can be very stressful. And the demands of so many

people using the same facilities can lead to things breaking down, so that city councils have to budget for constant maintenance and city dwellers may be taxed more.

The pressure of large numbers of people living in a limited space also makes the need for both peace and security an important concern. This is being addressed in different ways. Besides installing more efficient traffic-control systems and passing antinoise laws, some cities have established car-free zones that have made shopping areas and residential streets safer and more pleasant places; the absence of traffic reduces both noise and air pollution.

Local governments and action groups are doing much to tackle the challenges of urban living. Initiatives such as Neighborhood Watch encourage neighbors to keep an eye out for any suspicious behavior and to work closely with the local police force to fight crime. International movements such as Agenda 21 (see right column) are working to help rekindle the close-knit, healthy, "village" atmosphere that once existed in many towns and cities.

Congested traffic in cities poses perhaps the most serious challenge of all. According to research at Lancaster University in England, up to 15 million citizens in the United Kingdom could be suffering from health problems caused by exhaust fumes. A study by the British National Society for

AGENDA 21
At the Rio Earth Summit in 1992, 179 nations signed the Agenda 21 agreement—a plan for sustainable development "to meet the needs of the present without compromising the ability of future generations to meet their needs." Examples of Agenda 21 initiatives are

▶ *Planting community woodlands to ensure plenty of green spaces in urban areas and to combat the amount of carbon dioxide entering the atmosphere.*

▶ *Cleaning up canals and waterways to eliminate water pollution and provide alternative means of transportation.*

▶ *Establishing exchange systems in which community members can barter their skills instead of using cash. (This is an effective way of rejuvenating poor areas.)*

▶ *Encouraging carpools and ride sharing to reduce road congestion and pollution.*

▶ *Delivering organic vegetables to individuals every week.*

▶ *Setting up community compost sites so that vegetable and garden waste can be recycled and used to benefit the community rather than discarded in landfill sites.*

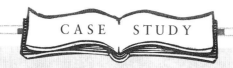

A Restless Retiree

A life-changing event like retirement can mean spending more time at home, and the place of residence may then take on greater importance. When a retired married couple disagrees about where they want to live and what they want to get from their environment, the rancor can cause serious problems in their relationship.

Megan retired recently from her busy job as a legal secretary in a large city. She and her husband, Tom, have lived in the same house for their entire married life, but now that they have both retired, they are not sure what they want to do. Megan grew up in the country and has always dreamed of retiring to a more rural area where she could tend a garden and spend time walking and bird-watching. Tom, who worked as a taxi driver, wants to stay in the city because he feels he would miss the variety of movies, as well as the local bars that fulfill his need for social company. They have been having increasingly frequent arguments about their future, and Megan is beginning to suffer from migraine headaches.

WHAT DID MEGAN DO?

Megan consulted her doctor to make sure that her migraines were not a symptom of something more serious. The doctor told her that her health problems were possibly stress related and that she and Tom should see a counselor to get help in resolving their differences. The counselor encouraged Megan to think more laterally about their problems and try to understand Tom's insecurities about leaving his old way of life. He also advised her to consider if she might be remembering her childhood through a rosy haze. Since analyzing her feelings and discussing future goals with Tom, Megan is now able to look for common ground to satisfy both of their needs.

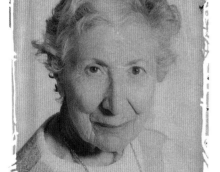

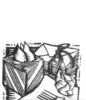

COMMUNICATION
Not discussing feelings and worries can make a couple drift further apart, resulting in health problems.

LIFESTYLE
Disputes about the way of life a couple should adopt in the future can have far-reaching effects on their relationship.

EMOTIONAL HEALTH
Unresolved difficulties and worries about the future can affect physical health, causing headaches and sleep disturbances.

Action Plan

LIFESTYLE
Look for activities and hobbies that combine town and country pursuits. Take time to enjoy each other's company and make plans for facing the future together.

EMOTIONAL HEALTH
Make an effort to discuss problems and concerns as they arise. Get adequate relaxation to relieve symptoms of stress.

COMMUNICATION
Be honest with each other about fears and ambitions and work to resolve issues before they become major problems.

HOW THINGS TURNED OUT FOR MEGAN

Counseling helped Megan to realize that both she and Tom were feeling insecure about retirement. After much discussion, they compromised and moved to a smaller house with a garden not far from their old home. Megan can be outdoors more, and Tom can enjoy his pastimes. They have regular days out together and often meet friends at a neighborhood restaurant. Megan's headaches have stopped, and they are both more content.

Clean Air revealed that traffic pollution worried 30 percent of the people surveyed a great deal, and many urban dwellers cite traffic noise and pollution as major factors in their decision to move out of the city, although the countryside is not without its own pollution problems (see page 74).

It is usually unnecessary to own a car in a large city because of an abundance of public transportation, but many people do keep one for convenience and for getting out of the city on weekends. This has contributed even more to pollution and congestion. A company in Seattle has had some success with a partial solution. It is a share-rental system for which people pay a fee to join and then pay a low hourly rate for the time they actually use a car. As many as 200 people can share 15 cars, and the savings over owning an automobile are enormous.

Urban noise levels are also of great concern to many persons, and while vehicles have been getting cleaner in their use of fuel, there has been little focus on their becoming quieter. In urban areas some 63 percent of people are exposed to nighttime noise levels above those recommended by the World Health Organization (WHO), and during the day 52 percent of people suffer noise that exceeds the WHO levels. Most of this disturbance is reported as traffic noise.

As working patterns continue to change and more people are able to work at home, commuter traffic may be reduced. There is also pressure for freight to be redirected back onto the rail network, which would lessen road use by trucks. Currently the best defense against environmental noise is the thorough insulation of houses, which not only cuts down on noise from the outside environment but also saves energy.

Stress is another factor in urban living that can lead to health problems. Crowded streets, irritated commuters, and busy stores in which long waits are inevitable are just a few of the things that contribute to high levels of frustration in urban dwellers and cause anxiety, depression, or feelings of overwhelming pressure. However, in most cities therapies that promote relaxation are readily available to counter the stresses of urban life. These include yoga, massage, and aromatherapy. It is also worth remembering that rural life can cause stress too, although the triggers may be different. For example, isolation or lack of stimulation

COPING WITH CROWDS

Many people find coping with crowds a particularly stressful aspect of city life. Being caught in a traffic jam or on a crowded train or bus with poor ventilation and minimal personal space can be particularly unpleasant; in some people it can cause feelings of claustrophobia or panic attacks. To help yourself cope more effectively with stressful situations, try this relaxation technique.

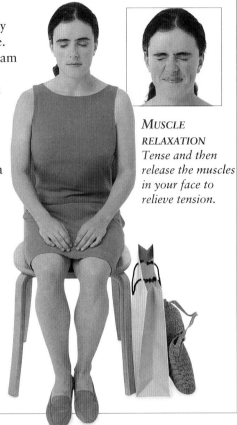

MUSCLE RELAXATION
Tense and then release the muscles in your face to relieve tension.

DEEP BREATHING AND VISUALIZATION
Either seated or standing, close your eyes and concentrate on breathing deeply and slowly. Then visualize yourself in calm and peaceful surroundings.

can cause boredom, loneliness, and anxiety. Many of the stress problems in the city that relate to emotional and behavioral issues might be addressed by adopting a more positive or accepting outlook, rather than relying on resolution through a change of environment.

RURAL LIVING

The country and suburbs are seen by most people as healthier and safer places to live than the city, imbued with qualities considered essential to a fulfilling life, including more psychological and physical space. In a poll taken in 1989, 72 percent of people said they would prefer to live outside a city. But the reality in the United States is that nearly 74 percent of the population now lives in urban areas. However, this may be changing. Although fewer people today work directly on the land than ever before in our history, more persons are choosing to leave the city and settle in a more rural area if their working life permits. It is estimated that in the United States and Great Britain approximately 300 people have moved away from cities every day for the past 20 years.

Flight relief
Researchers at the University of Sydney, Australia, have developed a window that closes automatically when a plane approaches a house located under a flight path. The window has built-in software to identify approaching aircraft noise before the human ear can detect it. Once the plane has passed, the window opens again.

Houses in the country and suburbs are often less expensive than in the city, and there is less pollution and usually less stress. The suburbs seem particularly attractive to city dwellers who have young children. The perception is that children can grow up enjoying greater independence because there is more open space for playing, less traffic, and less crime than in a city. However, many older children become bored by the limited choice of activities in the suburbs and the need always to be driven somewhere. Both rural and suburban life are changing, and it is important to be aware of negative aspects in either place that can have an impact on your health and happiness.

Problems in rural areas

The levels of chemicals used in modern farming practice can pollute the surrounding countryside. Pesticides, fertilizers, and intensive methods of raising stock create toxins not found in urban areas, and they are potentially just as damaging to health as city pollutants. Organophosphates and silage effluent leaking from farms into streams and underground water sources have caused serious pollution and health problems; so has crop spraying. Agricultural practices are increasingly responsible for the contaminants found in wells and community water supplies, and nitrous oxide released by the spreading of livestock waste as fertilizer on fields is known to pollute the air.

Traffic congestion can be almost as big a problem outside the city as in it. Rural and suburban people rely on their cars far more than city dwellers do and often commute long distances with only one person per car. Distances may be too great for bicycling, and public transportation is usually limited. Also, long distances between built-up areas can make traveling costly, and those people who do not have their own means of transportation may feel isolated.

Congestion can be a particular problem in small towns where streets are narrow. The increasing number of city dwellers visiting villages in rural farm and seaside areas each weekend also contributes to a growing traffic problem on rural roads. Building new roads is not necessarily a viable solution because they change the character of the countryside and contribute to pollution.

Some cities and midsized towns have tried to cope with traffic congestion by providing bicycle paths or street lanes that commuters can use during the week and recreationists can take advantage of on weekends. Although many such lanes may be seeing limited use at present, the hope is that more people will use them in the future.

In the United States many areas of outstanding natural beauty, including several national parks, are currently under threat from ever-increasing traffic. Proposals are being considered for limiting the number of visitors each year and for establishing parking areas outside the facilities and moving people in and out with buses or trams.

Rural unemployment is an ever-increasing problem too, often outstripping the unemployment problems in cities. It can affect young people especially, and the lack of facilities such as movie theaters and youth clubs for this age group can add to their frustration and boredom and possibly lead to crime. Demonstrations and protests in the United Kingdom, France, the United States, and other countries have highlighted the extent of distress among farmers and other rural dwellers today. Fluctuating agricultural prices and pressure to do away with traditional farming methods have contributed to increased levels of stress and uncertainty facing rural communities.

If you are considering moving from a city to a rural or suburban area, you may find it worthwhile first to reassess all the ramifications of changing your environment. Transportation options, available services and facilities, and health issues are all important factors to consider when weighing the pros and cons of such a move.

COUNTRY CONGESTION
Many areas of natural beauty are being threatened by overwhelming numbers of people and cars. For example, the wild grandeur of Stonehenge, near Salisbury, England, has been compromised by the proximity of a major highway. Increasing numbers of visitors and acts of vandalism have led to the site being fenced off from the public.

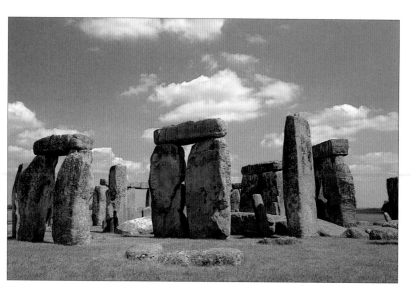

Selecting A Home Site

To enjoy the healthiest possible environment for living, consider the way your home is sited, how much light it receives, and the level of pollution it is exposed to.

When deciding where to live, look for factors that can help you achieve a healthier, safer, and more economical lifestyle and try to avoid such inherent problems as poor natural light or proximity to pollution sources—for example, major roads or industrial plants. Some undesirable aspects of existing buildings can be remedied, but if you are choosing a home or land to build on, the more beneficial the location and design of the house, the better.

Paying close attention to the environment of a new residence can save frustration in the future. It is worth walking around the area you are thinking of moving to and asking real estate agents and neighbors about the diversity and availability of services and leisure and cultural activities. Of course, you also have to consider practical matters, such as the area's proximity to your job, friends, and family.

It is possible these days to find or build a house that is environmentally sound and fits well into its surroundings and at the same time provides you with a comfortable home that benefits your health. All you need are well-thought-out preparations and a carefully chosen site.

Rules and regulations

Even if you do not plan to build, you should investigate local planning regulations. These are intended to protect the existing environment and control future development in the locality. Most districts are divided into zones that keep industrial areas separate from residential ones. Before buying land on which to build a house, you should seek professional advice because in many areas, planning laws can be complex. If you are considering an existing building, you should conduct a thorough search to make sure there are no restrictions to its access and to establish what extent of development would be permitted on the property. You should think twice about buying a residential property close to a zone designated for commercial or industrial development because you could find yourself living next to a shopping mall, industrial park, or office complex.

Public rights-of-way and the location of public lands should always be taken into account because they can affect your property too. Local authorities can develop city-owned property in any way they see fit for the needs of the community, which would include recreational facilities or playgrounds. They also have the right to purchase any adjoining land, so it is worth checking to see if any future developments are planned in the area. Maps that show public access and common land are usually available for viewing at the county land office or public library.

ECO-FRIENDLY VILLAGES
In many parts of the world, developers are designing communities in which health, use of renewable energy and building materials, and minimal impact on the environment are major considerations. One such development is Ecolonia, near Amsterdam. It has 101 family dwellings that make use of solar energy, recyclable materials, and systems that save water.

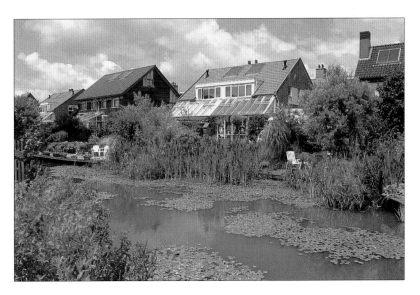

MAKING THE MOST OF SUNLIGHT IN YOUR HOME

If you are building your own home or buying a new one, take a close look at all the features of the site. To gain the most from natural sunlight, the rooms used most frequently, especially during the day, should face the path of the sun, while rooms that are used infrequently or only at night can be located in parts of the house that receive less sunlight.

North

A room used for laundry needs little natural light; a playroom should face a direction in which it receives more sunlight.

Bedrooms can be situated in almost any part of the house, but morning light is especially good for them.

West

East

Utility room

Storage

NO SUN ZONE

Sunset

Sunrise

Living room

SUN ZONE

Breakfast room

Play room

Conservatory/Kitchen

Bedrooms

*NATURAL LIGHT
In this diagram rooms in the sun zone get the most light and are used most often; the ones to the north receive little or no sun and less frequent use.*

A kitchen or conservatory should be positioned where the maximum amount of natural light enters the house.

South

PROTECTED AREAS

Areas subject to special planning controls may have restrictions that can affect private property. The most common of these controlled areas are

▶ *state and national forests and parks*

▶ *nature preserves*

▶ *areas in which threatened or endangered species are protected*

▶ *environmentally sensitive areas*

▶ *regions in which water is scarce*

▶ *green belts*

▶ *national historic sites*

▶ *sites of archaeological interest*

Pollution and other considerations

When choosing a site, it is important to take into account any pollution that might affect your family's health, such as noise and fumes from roads and highways

Noise can be a big problem, disrupting sleep and causing considerable stress. Industrial parks, gas stations, factory farms, an airport flight path, and even leisure facilities, such as a go-cart track or a skeet-shooting range, can be a big noise nuisance.

Air pollution can affect respiratory health, and in some areas the presence of radon in the local bedrock can cause a variety of health risks that should be considered (see page 57). Street lighting in towns and cities may be disrupting as well, especially if it prevents or delays sleep.

If your home is exposed to the sun, you can take advantage of it by installing a solar system. Today these can meet a number of energy functions, including heating or cooling the house, heating water for the house or a swimming pool, and providing electricity

and/or refrigeration. You can also take advantage of the sun by adding on a green-house or sunroom (conservatory). After the initial outlay, you will save on heating bills and benefit from increased humidity, especially helpful where desert air or indoor heating make the air in the home very dry. Adding insulated shades or draperies will help conserve the heat at night.

Another important factor to think about is whether your home is sheltered from or exposed to prevailing winds. If you are vulnerable to harsh elements, one solution is to plant a windbreak of trees or tall shrubs. Depending on where your home is located, different aspects have to be considered. For example, in warm climates it is better to choose a site at a higher elevation or facing the sea in order to benefit from breezes. In climates where there is intense winter cold, however, it is better to choose a sheltered site protected by trees or other buildings that will provide protection in winter and shade in summer. It is worth remembering

THE HEALTH OF TREES

Research conducted by Dr. Glynn Percival of the Scottish Agricultural College in Ayrshire has shown how modern living can be just as stressful for trees as for humans. Birch and cypress, for example, are particularly prone to salt damage from winter treatment of roads and badly aerated soils. Specimens growing in urban environments were found to have an average life span of just 32 years, compared to 150 years typical of the same trees growing in the country. Hardier species are a better choice for street planting because their roots can survive with less oxygen. Planting the right trees can help maintain greener urban environments.

that prevailing winds can also bring atmospheric pollution; in this case trees and shrubs offer both shelter and a filtration system for pollutants. Valleys, especially in warmer climates, can be potential traps for pollution (see page 38), so bear this in mind if you suffer from respiratory problems.

Choosing a home that is near your workplace is beneficial in several ways, especially if you have to commute by car. Not only does daily time on the road add to pollution, but it can also cause stress and subtract from time spent with your family or in leisure pursuits. Commuting accounts for a substantial portion of household expenditures for many people. Living within walking or bicycling distance of work can save money and also keep you fit, as well as contribute in a small way to reducing traffic congestion and pollution. If living close to your workplace is not possible or desirable, consider using other transportation options, such as trains, buses, or a car pool to ease the burden on the environment.

Ecological concerns

The ecology of a site is a fairly good indicator of the health of an area. A plenitude of trees and shrubs plus birds and other wildlife can be a sign that the environment is relatively healthy and that pollution and noise disturbance are minimal.

If the property surrounding your home is large enough to incorporate trees and shrubs, these will act as useful windbreaks and noise barriers and provide food and habitats for wildlife. There are even a few plants—sunflowers and fescue grass, for example—that can help mop up toxins. These have been used in reclaiming degraded or derelict urban areas that were previously contaminated by industry.

KEEPING ROOTS AT A SAFE DISTANCE

Some trees have extensive root systems that can damage utility pipes, sidewalks, and even the structural foundations of a building. This could result in costly repair work, as well as threaten the life of the tree. Before choosing a tree to plant, find out how far away from your home you should plant it to avoid future damage. The table below is a guide to the approximate safe distances for some popular trees.

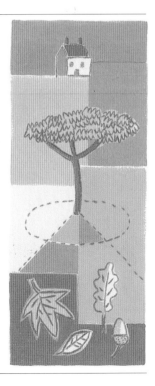

ROOT GROWTH OF COMMON TREES			
Poplar	20 feet	Magnolia	15 feet
Elm	20 feet	Horse chestnut	15 feet
Oak	20 feet	Cedar	12 feet
Willow	20 feet	Locust	12 feet
Beech	20 feet	Birch	12 feet
Ash	15 feet	Magnolia	12 feet
Sycamore	15 feet	Hawthorn	10 feet
Sugar maple	15 feet	Pine	10 feet

CHANGING YOUR HOME

Whether building or renovating a house, your choice of materials and methods can have a positive effect, not just on your own health but also on the local and wider environments.

GOOD BUILDING MATERIALS

When building or renovating a home, consider using natural, renewable, nontoxic, and energy-conserving materials, such as

▶ *insulated concrete for the foundation*

▶ *insulation made from recycled cellulose*

▶ *stone, adobe, straw bale, structured insulated panels, rammed earth, or stucco for exterior walls*

▶ *plaster or wood for interior walls*

▶ *wood, ceramic tile, granite, slate, or marble for floors and countertops*

▶ *carpeting made of wool, coir, or jute*

Housing needs change over a lifetime. For example, the arrival of a baby, older children leaving home, an elderly relative coming to live with you, or a new job in another part of the country could mean that a house move is necessary. You may be part of the population that has become increasingly mobile over the past several decades. During the 1960s people in America changed homes on average every seven years. By the end of the 1980s they were moving far more frequently, in some cases as often as every eight months. It is reasonable to assume, therefore, that at some point most home owners will move. Or they might decide to build an extension onto their existing home.

If you decide to make some renovations, consider hiring an architect or builder who can help you include in your plans innovations that conserve energy and are kind to the environment in other ways (see pages 80–81). Such a professional will also be familiar with building codes in your area and can help you acquire the necessary permits, as well as locate the materials you want.

BUILDING OR RENOVATING YOUR OWN HOME

When building or renovating a home, you have an opportunity to select materials that are environmentally friendly. Just keep in mind that all building projects are subject to strict regulations and inspections that can be complex, so it is advisable for even the most proficient do-it-yourself person to seek professional advice and guidance from an architect or building contractor at the planning stages. Although employing a professional will cost money, your project will stand a much better chance of success. You

Origins

Frank Lloyd Wright was one of the first 20th-century architects to promote ecological awareness and planning in architecture. He designed houses to integrate with their settings in such a natural way that they appeared to rise organically from the surrounding landscape.

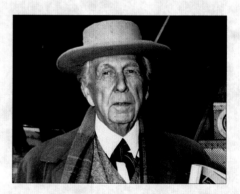

FRANK LLOYD WRIGHT (1869–1959)
A strong inventive voice within mainstream modern architecture, Frank Lloyd Wright championed a more ecologically sensitive style of building.

may even save money in the long run because architects and builders know where to find the best materials and are eligible for discounts. Also, their expertise may prevent you from making some costly mistakes.

Finding an architect or builder
The best way to find an architect is by personal recommendation. Talking to previous clients about their experiences can yield a reasonable insight into the way an architect

works. If this proves difficult, check around town for projects that are underway. Any professional will have a sign posted on a job with his or her name and phone number. You can contact this person and ask for references or talk to the people who commissioned the work you saw in progress.

Word of mouth is also a good way to find a builder; you should look for one who has relevant experience and is sympathetic to your needs. For instance, working on a stucco house demands a different set of skills than building a brick structure.

Ask a builder if you can view examples of his or her work to see if it is similar to the plans you have in mind. Also, find out from previous clients if their job was completed in a timely fashion; if it was supposed to be finished in six weeks and dragged on for six months, you may want to consider another contractor. Talk as well to the builder's subcontractors—electricians and carpenters, for example—to make sure they have been paid. Some contractors overextend themselves and don't pay all their suppliers or subcontractors, leaving the home owner to cope with the aftermath.

Home inspections
When buying a home, you should have a building inspection carried out before you commit yourself financially. Inspections are usually required by mortgage lenders, but even if you do not need financing, they are an important precautionary measure. The typical inspection will include comments on many key aspects concerning the condition of the building and property. The report will reveal evidence of settling, dry rot, leaking pipes, basement dampness, termites, roofing problems, structural damage, violations of local building codes, poor repair jobs, and other conditions that could affect the safety and value of the property. You may also want to commission a land survey that will establish the dimensions of the site and clearly define its boundaries.

BUILDING MATERIALS
The average home can take more than 20 years to consume as much energy as was used in the manufacture of its building materials. It is thus environmentally better to use as many recycled and renewable materials as you can for a new building or home improvement. When renovating, salvage and reuse as much material as possible from your own house. If you are using a building contractor to do the work, stress this point. Usually very little care is taken with demolition because it takes longer and is more expensive in the short term.

It also makes sense to select materials that will make your home more energy efficient. These include double-paned windows and

continued on page 82

CREATIVE USES FOR SALVAGED ITEMS

Before you throw away old or broken household items, consider ways in which they might be adapted to make useful or decorative features around your home.

▶ *Salvaged lumber can be used to construct garage shelving, a garden structure, or a planter. If it's weathered, it might make attractive paneling for a kitchen or den.*

▶ *A broken wheelbarrow can be propped up in the garden and filled with a variety of flowers.*

▶ *A deep bathtub can be buried in the garden and turned into a pond.*

▶ *An old cabinet can be refinished and used as detached open shelving if its doors are removed.*

HEALTH HAZARDS TO WATCH OUT FOR

Having a house inspected before committing to buying it will identify any problems that could be hazardous to your health or affect the value and safety of the house. The seller can be required to correct problems before the sale is complete.

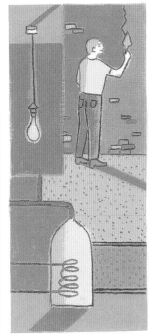

BUILDING PROBLEM	HEALTH IMPLICATION
Asbestos	Old walls, ceilings, and roofing could contain loosened asbestos. If inhaled, it can cause severe lung disorders.
Inadequate ventilation near gas stoves or heaters	Dangerous levels of carbon monoxide and other gases may build up. These fumes can cause nausea, headaches, and fatigue and can be fatal at high levels of exposure.
Old plumbing	The pipes in older houses often contain lead, which can leach into the water supply, causing fatigue, irritability, stomach pains, and headaches.
Termites	A severe termite problem will require that your entire home be treated with chemicals and that affected beams or siding be replaced.
Old paint	Old paint can be lead based or contain other toxic chemicals.
Dry rot	The chemicals used for treatment may give off toxins for up to two years.

The Environmental Architect

A well-planned home will meet both our physical and emotional needs and be sensitive to the environment at the same time. The goal of an environmental architect is to balance all three of these requirements.

Roof insulation

Heat reflectors

Pipe lagging

Insulated wall covering

KEEPING THE HEAT IN YOUR HOME
Insulating your home makes financial and ecological sense. Attic insulation prevents heat loss through the roof; pipe lagging maintains the temperature in the hot water system; reflectors behind radiators direct heat into a room; insulated wall covering keeps heat inside a room.

An environmental architect, whether commissioned to design a new house or adapt an existing one, seeks to match a building to the requirements of the client in a way that safeguards the environment. Using recycled materials or renewable ones from sustainable sources, the architect will try to create a healthy, attractive living environment in which energy consumption, waste production, and pollutants are kept to a minimum while comfort and energy conservation are maximized.

ENVIRONMENTAL ARCHITECTURE

Environmental architecture took hold during the self-sufficiency movement of the 1960s and evolved further in the wake of the oil crisis of the 1970s, which made energy conservation and efficiency a priority for many people. In the 1980s and 1990, growing awareness of such environmental problems as global warming, overconsumption of fossil fuels, and other aspects of human-kind's impact on the world's ecology led to an increasing demand for architecture that puts sustainability, as well as comfort, attractiveness, and affordability, at the heart of building design. Eco-friendly architecture is recognized by governments and corporations as one of the many paths toward the

fulfillment of the Agenda 21 obligations—as agreed to at the Rio Earth Summit in 1992 (see page 71).

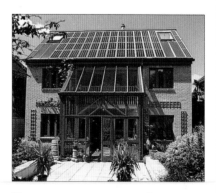

ECO-FRIENDLY HOUSE IN OXFORD
This solar-powered house in England, designed by architect Susan Roaf, produces an excess of electricity, which it puts back into the national grid.

What are the aims of an environmental architect?
Designing simple, attractive, and comfortable shelters that do not harm the earth is the general goal of environmental architects, and they strive to dovetail these parameters with the needs of their clients.

It is likely that you will be asked some personal questions before an architect plans your new home. You will be encouraged to talk about yourself, describing your work, hobbies, family activities, and leisure pursuits, as well as the budget you have for your project. The architect will also want to know what your requirements are for the garden.

An environmental architect regards your house and garden as an interconnected ecosystem and will design for a cyclical flow of air, water, waste products, and heat throughout the whole project. Energy and waste products will be recycled as much as possible.

Low maintenance and self-sufficiency are also major goals. Home owners shouldn't have to depend completely on electricity and other energy sources to stay healthy and comfortable and prevent disasters like frozen pipes.

Why is environmental architecture a healthy option?
People who have specific health concerns can especially benefit from the expertise of an environmental

architect. For someone who suffers from eczema or other allergies, for instance, an environmental architect will choose building materials that are nonallergenic and textiles and furnishings largely devoid of synthetic fibers or finishes that give off volatile organic compounds, which are likely to exacerbate allergies. He or she will also choose water-based paints and varnishes that do not give off toxic fumes.

There is more to be gained from environmental architecture than personal benefits. Creating an eco-friendly home makes individuals more aware of and responsible for the effects that their lifestyle and surroundings have on their health and the wider world.

How does an environmental architect work?

An environmental architect will first compile a profile of the needs of the client, based on initial discussions. He or she will then produce a design that meets as many of these needs as possible. For example, a young couple who work full-time and have little spare time for household maintenance or gardening might want a house that would require minimum upkeep. The interior would have built-in labor-saving features; the garden would be planted with drought-resistant perennials, trees, and shrubs that need only minimal maintenance; and fuel requirements would be met by an energy-efficient system. The house would be built in such a way that its owners could add new technologies as they are developed. Equally important, however, the house would offer a relaxing, peaceful space for escaping the tensions of working life.

A house designed for an active gardener and environmental enthusiast with plenty of time would be different in some respects. It would probably incorporate labor-saving devices and energy-efficient systems but might also include gray-water recycling and possibly a series

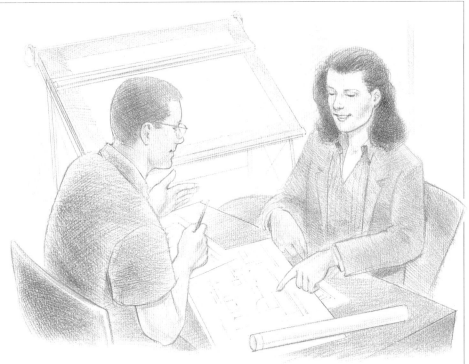

of ponds that would attract wildlife. A conservatory might be included for growing seedlings and exotic plants and would also be part of the solar heating system of the house. Composting would be part of a comprehensive waste management system. The house would ideally face south, and the roof would contain photovoltaic panels to provide electricity; a basement might include a cold-storage area for root vegetables.

Is environmental architecture cost-effective?

Some materials and technology may be more expensive than conventional ones initially, but a sustainable design is cost-effective in terms of energy efficiency and economical maintenance. By some estimates, just one eco-friendly house can reduce pollution by 500,000 pounds every 30 years! And 30,000 fuel-free homes could replace one nuclear plant.

The typical materials for environmental architecture are generally sturdy and disaster and fire resistant and should therefore see a longer life than those used for a conventional building. Environmental architects usually strive for affordability so that more people will be willing and able to use their designs.

ECO-FRIENDLY BLUEPRINTS
An environmental architect will draw up detailed plans and specifications for you to inspect, comment on, and approve before any work commences.

WHAT YOU CAN DO AT HOME

Draft-proofing and insulating your home can save energy and money. Insulation at least 6 inches thick in the attic alone can save 20 to 35 percent in energy costs each year. One especially eco-friendly form of insulation is cellulose fiber made from recycled newsprint. Other simple ways to cut energy costs include putting lagging on hot-water pipes to keep water warm; fitting draft blockers (foam plates) behind light switches and electrical outlets; clearing clutter away from windows to admit sunlight for warming rooms naturally; putting aluminum foil or thermal sheathing material behind radiators to bounce heat back into the room; installing double- or triple-glazed windows and hanging lined draperies or shades to prevent heat from escaping rooms at night; and covering windows with reflective window film to deflect indoor heat back into the room.

Creating a buffer wall for noise

If you live on a busy street, are near an industrial area, or have noisy neighbors, creating some kind of buffer zone can reduce noise. Despite being expensive to build, a wall is effective for absorbing sound, provided it is designed and built for the purpose; otherwise noise may simply bounce off of it. This can be mitigated somewhat by planting shrubs in front of the wall or by constructing a wall from a mixture of building materials to create texture; a wall of stone combined with bricks or salvaged masonry will absorb noise more effectively than a smooth wall and can make an interesting architectural statement as well. Highway engineers now incorporate ridges and indentations in concrete highway walls to absorb noise.

CAVE HOUSES
A vast ancient area of sandstone caves situated in Cappadocia, in the heart of Turkey, has long provided a unique form of housing for the local people. Many of the caves are still inhabited today, and some even provide simple accommodations for travelers.

structural insulated panels (SIP), which consist of expanded polystyrene sandwiched between two boards made of pressurized wood chips. Not only do these windows and panels save money on energy costs because they keep the interior temperature steady, but they also reduce noise from outside the building dramatically.

If you are doing the renovation yourself, take precautions, such as wearing a mask, to protect yourself from harmful toxins in the materials you remove. There could be asbestos in some of the building materials or lead in the paint. You should also cover yourself completely if you are removing fiberglass insulation, then remove your clothing and wash it separately.

When you use an environmental architect, he or she will design your project using as many renewable materials as possible. The most familiar of these are adobe, wood, stone, brick, slate, glass, plaster, and cement. Some newer or rediscovered materials include rammed earth, straw bale, and recycled bottles or tires for walls and recycled cellulose, newsprint, cardboard, and magnesium oxide bubbles for insulation.

Wood is one of the healthiest building materials. It is a natural regulator of the indoor climate, it breathes, and it stabilizes humidity, absorbs sound, and filters and purifies the air. However, tree felling without adequate reforestation has vastly diminished wood supplies. You should avoid buying endangered hardwoods, such as mahogany and teak; these also require huge amounts of fuel for transportation. Instead, choose hardwood and softwood trees that

are not under threat—oak, ash, and pine are three examples. Strong and durable, they are ideal for doors, furniture, and flooring.

Stone is also a nonpolluting, structurally strong, and durable building material. It does have a couple of drawbacks, however: quarries disfigure the landscape, and high energy costs are involved in the quarrying, handling, and transporting of stone.

Glass is a versatile material made from natural and renewable sources, but its production requires a vast amount of energy and creates pollution. This can be offset a little bit by using recycled windows, which also save money, and floor tiles that are made of recycled glass.

Avoid the use of plastics as much as possible. They consume vast amounts of energy during production, some of it polluting, and they are made with nonrenewable petrochemicals. Also, many plastics are non-biodegradable and cannot be recycled. Some present health risks as well. Soft thermoplastics, such as polyvinyl chloride (PVC) and polyethylene, leak toxic chemicals when warmed or when they come in contact with food and beverages. If you have PVC pipes in your home that were manufactured before 1977, you should have them replaced because they are dangerous to health.

Although many of the devices you can install, such as photovoltaic cells that turn energy from sunlight into electrical power, can initially be expensive, their energy efficiency means that they will soon pay for themselves in savings from reduced electricity bills.

The age of your home

A renewed interest in traditional building materials, such as wood, stone, and brick, has highlighted the benefits of older houses. Modern buildings, although convenient and desirable in many respects, have a tendency to trap interior air, including toxins and other pollutants that can build up to potentially harmful levels. People are now realizing that chemicals inside homes and public buildings may be the source of unexplained illnesses, diseases, or allergies. It is as important to deal with these as it is to eat healthfully and exercise regularly.

To circulate enough fresh air in your home, open the windows for at least 10 minutes every day, even during winter. This will allow stale, polluted air to escape and fresh air to flow in. You will probably feel healthier as a result. While airing your home, turn down the thermostat so that energy is not wasted when the window is open.

ENERGY SYSTEMS IN THE HOME

Making use of the sun's energy is one of the most beneficial things you can do to make your house more environmentally sensitive because you will use less energy from fossil fuel sources. There are two kinds of solar energy systems—active and passive.

Active systems for residential use involve the installation of special collectors. These may be fluid collectors, which heat water (see box, right), or photovoltaic cells, which convert sunlight into electrical energy. Even where winter sunlight hours are limited, solar water heating has proved efficient enough to take the chill off water so that only minimal conventional heating is needed; for the rest of the year the systems provide plentiful hot water.

Photovoltaic (PV) cells operate with concentrated sunlight and work best when mounted on a tracking device. Their efficiency is only about 15 percent under the best of circumstances, so they are practical only in the sunniest parts of the country.

You do not have to install solar panels to benefit from the sun's energy, however; you can use passive solar collection. The south side of a building receives the most sunlight. At a very simple level, all windows on this side become solar collectors. If you have several large windows that face the sun, these will absorb heat into a room and reduce your need for conventional heating by up to 15 percent. This occurs because light energy that passes through windows is transformed into heat as it hits the interior walls and floors. The heat is then reflected off these surfaces within the room, and the windows then act like mirrors, bouncing back the energy to keep the heat in the room. To minimize heat loss through the windows, install double-glazed types and caulk them well. Use insulated shades or draperies to prevent heat loss at night.

Too much sunlight can be a problem during the summer months. Overhangs as part of the design on the south side of the house will at least partly shade the windows, and shutters or insulated draperies or shades will keep the sun out altogether during the hottest hours of the day.

HOW SOLAR ENERGY PROVIDES HOT WATER

The sun provides the earth with a vast amount of energy that can be harnessed in a clean and safe way, not only to heat or cool a home but also to provide hot water. Even in cooler climates where cloudy days are more numerous, solar panels are a good investment.

Hot water flows into the tank.

Cold water enters the tank, sinks to the bottom, and flows through the pipes and into the solar panel.

The solar panel heats the water, which automatically flows into the tank as hot water is used.

Cold water out

Hot water

Tank

Cold water

Cold water from the tank flows through the pipes to the solar panel.

SOLAR PANELS
Metal collector panels covered with glass or plastic are usually housed in shallow boxes and fixed in rows on a sun-facing roof or wall.

An ecologically designed house will recycle as many waste products as possible. This not only is environmentally smart but can also save money. Such a building recycles by-products, incorporating them back into the system at various stages, thereby creating cyclical energy flows within the ecosystem of the home and garden. A small-scale example of this is a compost heap (see page 87), which puts kitchen and garden waste to good use. A more elaborate approach is the recycling of household, or gray, water for use in the garden.

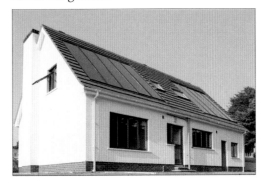

HARNESSING THE SUN'S ENERGY
This house in Northern Ireland has solar panels on the roof to collect energy from the sun's rays. Even in a cloudy climate, solar power can make a significant contribution to domestic energy requirements.

A Water Feature

A water feature near your home—a small pool, miniature waterfall, or bubbling fountain, for example—can have a significant effect on its dominant chi, or life energy, and add light, movement, and sound to the environment.

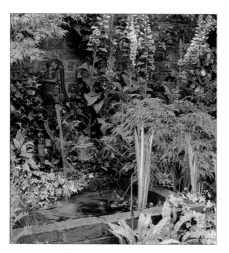

FOUNTAINS FOR ENERGY
Attractive in itself, a fountain prevents a pond from stagnating and makes the water more active, which creates an upward flow of chi.

In feng shui (see pages 104–112) water represents money because money flows through a community the way water flows through a landscape. Water also represents life and vitality; a water feature in your garden can help balance your home's chi. For instance, an overly energized site can be calmed with a small fish pond, or a very still and calm setting can be enlivened with a gushing waterfall or a fountain. If you do not live by a natural water feature,

installing a pond, fountain, or birdbath in your garden is a suitable alternative. These will also attract wildlife and give you an opportunity to grow water lilies and other kinds of water plants if you choose.

The best location for siting a water feature is in the southeast or east section of your garden. The southeast is believed to encourage creativity and communication and the east to promote activity and the realization of your dreams.

CREATING A MINI WATER GARDEN

If you have no room in your garden for a full-size pond, a half-barrel mini pond is a good solution. Place the barrel where desired and set it on bricks to let air circulate underneath and prevent the base from rotting. Coat the barrel with preservative and allow it to dry thoroughly, then line

it with thick black polyethylene, cover the bottom with pebbles, and fill it nearly full with water.

You can grow many plants in a water garden; miniature water lilies are especially pretty. These can be planted in a plastic basket and then lowered into the water.

MINI WATER GARDEN
Creating a small pond out of a half barrel is a quick and simple way to add an attractive water feature to any garden.

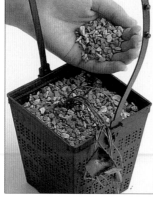

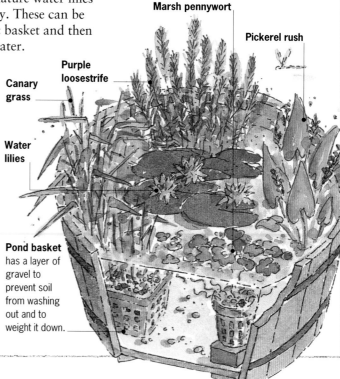

Marsh pennywort

Pickerel rush

Purple loosestrife

Canary grass

Water lilies

Pond basket has a layer of gravel to prevent soil from washing out and to weight it down.

1 *Plant water lilies in soil in a plastic basket; insert a slow-release fertilizer pellet near the roots.*

2 *Carefully top the soil with a layer of gravel or tiny stones to prevent the soil from being washed away.*

DESIGNING YOUR GARDEN

A well-designed garden can make a big contribution to a healthy home environment. Plants can reduce noise pollution, absorb pollutants, provide privacy, and reduce your stress levels.

Gardens have been an important aspect of life in many cultures throughout the centuries. They have served as places of tranquillity, recreation, and respite from the outside world, as well as spaces for growing food. If you do not have access to a garden, window boxes and potted plants can provide a few of the benefits. Gardens satisfy some basic psychological as well as physical needs. They bring pleasure and help people reduce their stress levels and express their creativity. Gardening can also be a good form of gentle physical exercise.

To get the most out of your garden, you should take into account the particular features of your plot—where there is shade or sun or exposure to wind and what type of soil predominates. You must also consider what sort of plants grow well in your area.

Ideally when planning a garden, it is advisable to take a full year to observe the effects of the environment in each season, such as the cycles of the sun, the prevailing winds, any sources of pollution, the average rainfall, and how well existing plants are thriving. Twelve months may seem like a long time to wait before getting started, but your patience will be rewarded. Careful observation and preparation not only will save you from potential mistakes but also will ensure that you ultimately enjoy a successful and satisfying garden.

LEARNING ABOUT YOUR GARDEN

Answering the questions below can help you to plan a successful garden.

▶ *What is the general soil type? Are there pH variations in different parts of the garden?*

▶ *What plants are indigenous to the area and what other species are commonly grown?*

▶ *What sort of garden pests are common in the area and how are they best controlled?*

▶ *What is the average annual rainfall?*

▶ *What are minimum and maximum temperatures for each season?*

▶ *In what gardening zone are you located?*

▶ *In which direction does each section of the garden face?*

▶ *Where does the household waste go?*

▶ *Where does the water supply come from?*

▶ *How high is the garden above sea level?*

▶ *From which direction does the prevailing wind come?*

TESTING FOR YOUR SOIL TYPE

The first stage in developing a successful garden is to determine your soil's texture and its degree of acidity or alkalinity. This will tell you what kind of plants you can grow successfully or how you need to amend the soil. The best way to identify soil texture is by rubbing a small amount in your hand. You can test the soil pH value with a kit available from garden centers. Mix a sample of soil with the kit's chemical solution; the color of the solution reveals the pH.

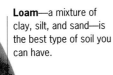

CHECKING SOIL TEXTURE
Clay soil feels fairly smooth and sticky; sandy soil feels dry and gritty.

Loam—a mixture of clay, silt, and sand—is the best type of soil you can have.

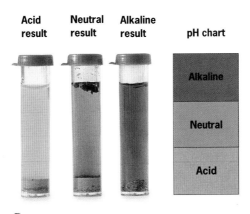

Acid result Neutral result Alkaline result pH chart

Alkaline

Neutral

Acid

COLOR TESTING KIT
Once the soil and chemical solution has stabilized, you can measure your soil type against the pH chart provided in the kit.

If you have moved to a new area, ask the neighbors, other local gardeners, and garden centers for advice. This will not only prevent you from making unsuitable choices of flowers, shrubs, and other plants but also help you get to know people in the community; you may even be given some cuttings or seedlings by neighborly gardeners to start you off. It is worth remembering that no two gardens are exactly alike—soil types and general conditions can vary over short distances—and you might have some success with plants that your neighbors have not considered trying.

COMMON DANGEROUS PLANTS

If you have young children, you should be aware of common plants that are poisonous. You may not necessarily want or need to remove these plants if they are already growing in your garden; pruning them so that they are out of reach of young children or explaining the dangers to older children may be sufficient.

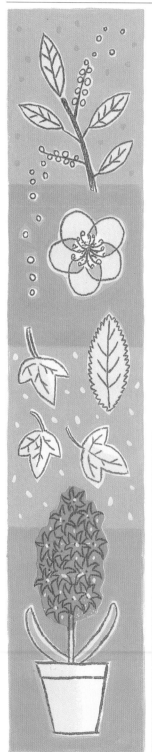

PLANT	POISONOUS PART	SYMPTOMS
Aconitum	All parts	Severe, possibly fatal, poisoning
Aesculus	All parts	Respiratory paralysis and mild gastrointestinal effects if eaten
Arnica montana	All parts	Internal pain, even death, if eaten; skin irritation if touched
Colchicum autumnale	All parts	Burning in throat, vomiting, followed by respiratory failure if eaten
Daphne mezereum	All parts	Severe poisoning if eaten; irritation of skin from sap
Delphinium ajacis	All parts	Nausea, vomiting, throat inflammation, skin itching if eaten
Dieffenbachia	All parts	Severe poisoning if eaten; irritation of skin from sap
Digitalis purpurea	All parts	Headache, convulsions, vomiting, and heart arrythmias if eaten
Euonymus	Berries	Diarrhea, vomiting, difficulty breathing, and stupor if eaten
Euphorbia cyparissias	All parts	Burning in mouth, vomiting, diarrhea, and stupor if eaten
Hedera helix	All parts	Irritation to sensitive skin; poisoning if eaten
Hyacinthus	All parts	Diarrhea if eaten; dermatitis from sap
Hydrastis canadensis	All parts	Hypertension, nausea, diarrhea, and difficulty breathing if eaten
Kalmia latifolia	Leaves, flowers	Mouth and stomach pain, nausea, diarrhea, blurred vision if eaten
Laburnum	All parts	Vomiting, drowsiness, headache, increased heartbeat if eaten
Ligustrum vulgare	Leaves, fruits	Vomiting, diarrhea, and liver damage if eaten
Lupinus	Seeds	Nausea, vomiting, and dizziness if eaten
Narcissus	Bulbs	Vomiting and convulsions if eaten; irritation to skin if handled
Nerium oleander	All parts	Nausea, vomiting, and diarrhea if eaten; skin reaction if handled
Prunus virginiana	Leaves, fruit pits	Vomiting, convulsions, difficulty breathing, loss of balance
Ruta graveolens	All parts	Mild poisoning; possible blistering of skin when handled
Taxus canadensis	All parts	Vomiting, diarrhea, dilated pupils, and low blood pressure if eaten
Wisteria	All parts	Nausea, vomiting, and headache if eaten

PLANNING YOUR GARDEN

When creating a design for your garden, it's a good idea to start with a scale plan of the whole plot on graph paper. Include all the boundaries; existing hedges and trees; any constructions, such as a garden shed or greenhouse; and pathways. Also mark on your plan any areas in the garden that are particularly shady or damp, as well as the places that receive the most sunlight.

Before you begin planting, think about what the main uses of your garden will be. If you have children, you may want a lawn or other open area where they can play safely, and you should exclude any poisonous plants (see opposite page). If you are elderly or disabled, you might need a low-maintenance garden, perhaps with raised beds to reduce the amount of bending down. If you intend to entertain and spend a lot of time in the garden, you will probably want seating areas, perhaps even a built-in barbecue.

If you wish to grow vegetables, you will have to decide on a sunny and convenient part of the garden for the plot; to grow herbs, chose a spot close to the house for easy access. You should also consider where to site the compost heap, which needs some sunlight in order to develop. It should not

DID YOU KNOW?

Vegetables and fruits start to lose their vitamins and other nutrients as soon as they are picked. Freshly picked home-grown produce is actually better for you than store-bought—and it tastes better too.

be too far from the house, or you may never use it. To keep the compost heap out of sight, plan a way to screen it. You can use shrubs, such as a hawthorn hedge; a trellis covered with a vine like clematis; or a wall. You may want to invest in a special compost bin (see below), which is more convenient than a heap.

If you need ground covers, common sense dictates using shade-tolerant plants, such as *Ajuga reptans* (bugleweed) or *Hedera helix* (English ivy), in shady areas and sun-loving, drought-tolerant plants, such as *Juniperus horizontalis* (creeping juniper) or *Coronilla varia* (crown vetch), in areas that receive plenty of sunshine. *Vinca* (periwinkle) can grow in either sun or shade. Once you are clear about your needs and have a plan drawn up, it is relatively easy to produce a garden that is both practical and attractive.

STEP-BY-STEP COMPOSTING

Making and using good compost is one of the best things you can do for your garden. Compost provides nutrients for the soil, keeps the soil moist, and invites earthworms—one of the most beneficial of common garden species because they drag nutrients from the surface into the soil. Making good compost is quite easy, and because it also reduces household waste going into landfills, it is environmentally sound.

COMPOST INGREDIENTS

Layer 4 Cover the heap with a heavy plastic sheet. This minimizes moisture loss and keeps out rainwater, which can make it too wet.

Layer 3 Add a layer of grass clippings or leaves, and then repeat layers 1 to 3 to speed up the rotting process.

Layer 2 Fork on top a layer of garden trimmings, such as old bedding plants and cuttings; add fruit and vegetable scraps.

Layer 1 Spread a thin layer of woody prunings on the ground as a base so that the heap is raised slightly, helping air to circulate.

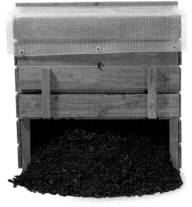

COMPOST CONTAINER
If you buy a compost bin, get one with ventilated walls, a lift-up panel to give you access to the compost, and a waterproof top.

TENDING COMPOST

Add compost ingredients in thin layers and intersperse moister materials with drier ones.

▶ *Use green materials that have a high nitrogen content; speed up the composting process with enzymes.*

▶ *Keep the compost insulated so the rotting process continues in winter.*

▶ *Keep the compost damp (not wet) because moisture encourages the materials to break down.*

Creating a

Wildlife Haven

A garden teeming with wildlife is not only an endless source of enjoyment for people of all ages but also a positive sign of a healthy environment; the presence of wild creatures often indicates minimal air and noise pollution.

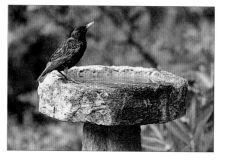

BIRDBATHS
A birdbath is a good way to attract a variety of birds to your garden.

Having birds, butterflies, beneficial insects, and amphibians in your garden creates a more balanced and peaceful environment. Many creatures fertilize the soil naturally or rid the garden of plant-damaging insects and diseases, thus reducing the need for artificial pesticides, which in turn benefits the environment. With careful preparation and planning, any garden, whether in an urban or country setting, can be transformed into a natural haven for a variety of wild creatures.

HOW TO ATTRACT WILDLIFE TO YOUR GARDEN

Retaining an old moss-covered wall can provide birds and other small creatures with natural shelter; the holes and crevices are ideal refuges, and the moss and weeds provide food in the form of seeds and insects.

An old tree stump can be used as a bird table. Attaching half coconuts that contain seeds will attract a variety of birds, some of them just passing through, many of them year-round residents who will attend the feast especially during the winter, when other food is usually scarce.

Unmowed grass in a sheltered, sunny area will act as a mini meadow, especially if you pepper it with native wildflowers; it will attract colorful hummingbirds, butterflies, and moths that feed off of nectar-rich flowers.

Trees and shrubs will act as natural sound barriers and provide birds with nesting sites and food in the form of berries.

Creating a pond with a mini waterfall in your garden will foster a tranquil and inviting atmosphere and also attract wildlife. You can introduce aquatic plants that will not only add beauty to the pond but also provide food and shelter. *Caltha*

palustris (marsh marigold, or cowslip), for instance, attracts bees and provides shelter for frogs and toads; tall irises are ideal for breeding dragonflies; and water lilies provide a pond with oxygen and help prevent stagnation. A pond will also attract birds, raccoons, and foxes, which all need water to drink and to wash in.

A WILDLIFE WONDERLAND
With just a small amount of effort, you can make any garden, large or small, attractive to myriad small creatures and birds.

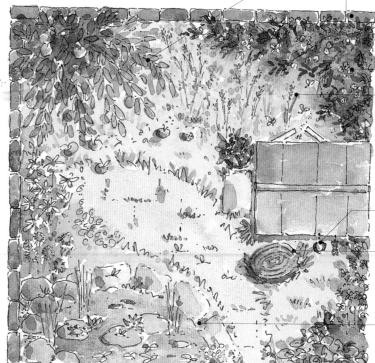

Fruit from trees provides food for birds.

A moss-covered wall provides food for insects.

Wildflowers attract butterflies.

Unmowed grass attracts insects and butterflies.

Coconuts filled with seeds provide extra food for birds.

A moss-covered tree stump makes a good bird table.

A pond attracts frogs, foxes, and raccoons.

PLANTING A NOISE-REDUCTION HEDGE

In addition to being an attractive feature of a garden, a hedge has many other advantages; it can be one of the most efficient forms of noise reduction, provide a filter for airborne pollution, and act as an effective privacy screen. If noise reduction is your priority, you need a broad hedge to make a significant difference. Choose a mixture of large-leaved and small-leaved evergreens; large-leaved plants suppress deeper sounds, while plants with smaller foliage eliminate higher tones. Use rhododendrons or azaleas as a foundation, include hollies, viburnum, or pyracantha for fall berries, and add cyprus or cedar for height.

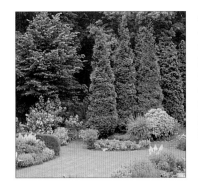

A LEAFY DEN
A high hedge around a garden not only provides privacy and reduces noise pollution but also creates a relaxing environment for you and a haven for wildlife.

BUILDING A SCREEN
If you have no room for a hedge, try a vine-covered trellis, which takes up very little space.

NOISE AND POLLUTION BARRIERS
Trees are good absorbers of pollution and noise, but you must be careful not to plant trees with large roots too close to the house because they can cause damage (see page 77).

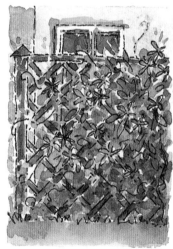

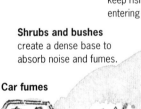

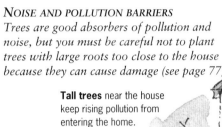

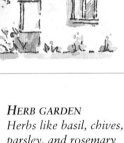

Tall trees near the house keep rising pollution from entering the home.

Climbing plants are an attractive way to cover a wall or a trellis. Evergreen species include akebia, jasmine, bougainvillea, creeping fig, and passionflower.

Shrubs and bushes create a dense base to absorb noise and fumes.

Car fumes

Sheltering belts of trees and shrubs can be grown along edges of the property exposed to roads or winds to reduce noise, pollution, and wind damage. Garden centers are usually happy to offer advice on plants that will be suitable for your particular garden and the locality in general.

When making choices for your garden, bear in mind your answers to the questions in the right margin on page 85; you should end up with a garden that not only is enjoyable to yourself but also benefits the wider local environment. It is always better, if you can, to grow indigenous trees, shrubs, wildflowers, and herbs because they are perfectly adapted to grow in your area and require less care and little or no fertilizer. Gardens that encourage beneficial insects and birds can also reduce the need for potentially harmful pesticides. Simple steps, such as installing a pond, providing a birdbath, and growing certain appealing plants, will attract wildlife to your garden.

VEGETABLE AND HERB GARDENS

Growing fresh vegetables and herbs for use in the kitchen is healthy and satisfying and also less expensive than buying organic produce from supermarkets or other suppliers. You can avoid using pesticides and thus be better able to safeguard your health and that of the environment. Even if you have a very small garden, you can still grow a few vegetables and herbs.

To reduce labor, you can plant perennial vegetables and herbs, such as chard, green onions, chicory, fennel, lovage, nasturtium, perennial kale, arugula, sorrel, rosemary, sage, salad burnet, tarragon, and thyme. You could also dedicate one or two areas to favorite annual crops, Examples are peas, garlic, green beans, onions, potatoes, tomatoes, lettuce and spinach. Fruit-bearing trees, like apple, cherry, lemon, and plum, can be included in your garden if there are favorable conditions.

HERB GARDEN
Herbs like basil, chives, parsley, and rosemary can be grown easily in special containers to provide you with a regular fresh supply for cooking.

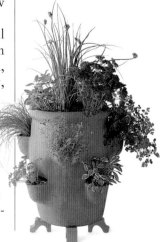

Herbs grow well among flower beds and in window boxes and flowerpots. A useful fact to remember is that the closer together you plant your vegetables and flowers, the less room there will be for weeds and the less maintenance your garden will need. Before planting, however, you should always check the size of mature plants and make sure that they will be happy growing in close proximity to others.

Certain plants are particularly suited to being grown together because the properties of one plant benefit the other. This is called companion planting. For example, it is beneficial to plant basil among tomatoes because the herb protects the tomatoes from aphids. French marigolds planted throughout a vegetable patch will deter whiteflies. Horseradish keeps pests away from potatoes; and garlic, onions, and chives protect carrots from carrot root flies.

Sheds and greenhouses

A shed is a practical addition to any garden if there is adequate space. It provides good storage for garden tools, bulbs, and seeds and a sheltered work pace for repotting plants or preparing seedlings. If there are children around, a shed allows you to keep potentially dangerous equipment locked up. It goes without saying that any chemicals, fertilizers, and pesticides should be locked out of the reach of children and used sparingly according to the manufacturer's directions. Better still, use organic methods so that you don't need them.

Tools should be cleaned after each use to prevent rust and dulling of blades. Electrical equipment, such as lawn mowers and trimmers, should also be cleaned and checked regularly to make sure that all parts are in good working order. Circuit breakers must

CHECKLIST

Power tools are safe to use in the garden as long as a few basic rules are observed. Try to keep them to a minimum, however, because they cause both air and noise pollution.

✔ *Always plug electrical equipment into a grounded outlet.*

✔ *Loop a cord over your shoulder and keep it behind you so you do not cut it while working.*

✔ *Do not use power tools outdoors when it is raining.*

✔ *Always turn off the power supply and remove the plug from the socket before adjusting or cleaning a tool.*

✔ *For safety's sake and to prolong the life of electrical equipment, have it checked regularly and serviced by an approved agent. Keep a close eye on cords for any signs of wear or damage.*

✔ *Use a heavy-duty extension cord that has a three-core rubber plug and a rubber socket. A cord should have the UL approval marked on it.*

✔ *Do not let children touch power equipment or distract you while you are working.*

A GARDEN NURSERY Greenhouses are perfect places to grow a variety of plants that require special care. When buying a greenhouse, choose the largest one you can; the larger the volume of air, the more controlled the growing environment. A greenhouse should be in full sunlight and away from overhanging trees.

be used with electrical equipment outdoors, and all plugs and sockets should have water-resistant hoods and be checked regularly.

Greenhouses are a considerable financial investment but are excellent for propagating seedlings and growing certain plants that require special conditions. To help control the amount of heat and moisture, a greenhouse needs at least one ventilator on each side of the roof and preferably one on each of the side walls. It also needs blinds on one or both sides of the roof, depending on how the greenhouse is situated.

It is important to keep a greenhouse meticulously clean to prevent the spread of plant diseases. On a regular basis you should wash all flowerpots and other equipment thoroughly and wash grime and algae from both sides of the greenhouse glass.

CHAPTER 4

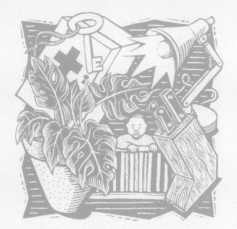

INSIDE YOUR HOME

More accidents occur in the home than anywhere else, and a large part of creating a healthy environment for yourself and your family is minimizing potential hazards. This chapter recommends some health and safety measures for the home, plus extra precautions for the elderly and young children. It also takes a look at how the effective use of light, space, and color can enhance comfort and offers a brief guide to the rudiments of feng shui.

HOUSEHOLD HAZARDS

No matter how healthy our homes are, there is always the potential for accidents to occur. Avoiding common household dangers is often a matter of being aware of possible problems.

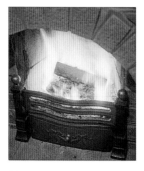

FIRE SAFETY
Logs crackling in the fireplace may be warming and attractive, but without a screen sparks can fly out of the grate and start a fire. Open fires are particularly dangerous if there are young children around. Always use a fireplace screen. A glass type is especially effective; not only does it fit snugly, but it prevents cold chimney air from entering the room when the fireplace is not in use.

Some 25 million home accidents occur in the United States each year as a result of faulty appliances or electrical connections, poor condition of floors, furniture, walls, or stairways, or inadequate lighting. Fire is one of the greatest risks; every precaution should be taken to prevent one from starting and to have an escape route should a fire take hold.

Many household fires can be prevented if electrical appliances and equipment are well maintained and used correctly. Frayed, cracked, or too tightly coiled cords or damaged wiring can cause shocks or fire. Always keep appliance cords in good condition and loosely coiled and make sure that plugs fit snugly into an outlet; otherwise, the socket may overheat and ignite. Two major causes of electrical fires in the home are overloaded outlets and extension cords. Extension cords alone are responsible for $1.3 billion in property damage and 6,300 serious injuries every year. (A new electronic power cord is now available that has specially shielded wiring and a "brain" that monitors the flow of electrical current and shuts it off when a problem arises.)

You can help reduce the risk of fire by not setting televisions, stereos, and other appliances too close to walls, which prevents air from circulating and can lead to overheating. You can also make sure that all light bulbs are of the correct wattage for a fixture or lamp; fixtures come with a tag that specifies the correct wattage. If in doubt, use a bulb of no more than 60 watts.

DO-IT-YOURSELF TIPS

Home improvement projects can be hazardous; paints and varnishes, for instance, contain toxins. Follow these tips to avoid injury and risks to health.

▶ *Ventilate the area in which you are working and wear protective clothing, such as a mask, goggles, and overalls, especially when working with oil-based paints or varnishes, sanding wood, or installing insulation.*

▶ *Always read the instructions carefully before using electrical tools.*

▶ *Keep electrical equipment away from water sources and take care with trailing cords.*

▶ *Make sure that a ladder is stable and strong enough to hold your weight.*

▶ *Avoid hammering nails into walls near switches, sockets, or through floors where there may be wires or water or gas pipes.*

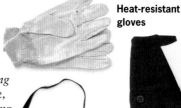

Heat-resistant gloves

Goggles

Antiglare glasses

Protective clothing

Face mask

SAFETY EQUIPMENT
Wearing protective goggles, a face mask, and protective clothing can prevent you from suffering an injury or a health problem.

FIRE PREVENTION AND SAFETY

There are simple measures you can take to protect yourself against fire and to escape safely in the event of a blaze.

▶ *Install smoke alarms in all areas of the house, not just the kitchen.*

▶ *Have an accessible exit from your home in addition to the front door.*

▶ *If you live in an apartment house, make sure you have good access to staircases and that emergency doors are unlocked.*

▶ *Make sure that you can open and climb out of at least one window in a room and, if it is above ground level, you own and know how to use a rope ladder.*

▶ *Keep keys to window locks and safety guards where you can easily locate them.*

▶ *Know the location of all fire extinguishers and how to use them.*

▶ *Keep all important documents in a fireproof safe or file box.*

▶ *Maintain all electrical and gas appliances in good working order.*

Gas heaters and fireplaces can also pose a fire risk; make sure there is a guard or screen over the flame, and keep children, pets, and clothing well away from it. Also, keep matches on a high shelf. Many fires are caused each year by children playing with matches.

Fumes

Because gas heaters release fumes, they should always be properly vented to the outside. For your safety, make sure that all gas furnaces and appliances are properly installed and regularly serviced. If gas should leak and the fumes build up, a spark could cause an explosion and fire.

Badly installed or faulty gas appliances can also produce large amounts of carbon monoxide, which can be lethal. At least 5,000 poisonings and 1,000 deaths occur in the United States each year from carbon monoxide; occurrences are especially common in mobile homes, where ventilation tends to be poor. If you suspect a gas leak or believe that an appliance may be faulty, call in a certified engineer immediately.

Another common source of carbon monoxide is the gas escaping from chimneys when wood is burned in a fireplace or wood stove. A badly designed or poorly maintained chimney can allow gases to blow back into the room. The buildup of residue in a dirty chimney can also catch fire and set the roof ablaze. Have your chimney cleaned at least every other year, more often if you use the fireplace frequently or burn soft woods like pine.

Attached garages, common in house plans today, are another household hazard. They can trap fumes from gasoline, oil, and exhaust pipes, which can then permeate the whole house. If your garage is attached, make sure that the connecting door to the house has a tight seal around the frame and remember to keep it closed at all times.

Chemical pollution indoors

It is a harsh fact of life that our homes and offices are often more polluted than the outdoor environment. This can be attributed to pollutants released by chemically treated building and furnishing materials, as well as products for cleaning and deodorizing. The increased use of insulating and draft-proofing materials also contributes to the problem because the chemicals cannot escape.

Products made from petrochemicals are the ones most likely to release toxins into the air, and if these vapors accumulate, they can become dangerous. Many such toxins are irritants that affect the mucous membranes in the eyes, mouth, throat, and lungs and may cause allergic skin reactions.

One particularly toxic chemical is formaldehyde, used as a binder and preservative in many building materials, such as particleboard, plywood, and pressed wood panels, and in soft furnishings, such as rugs, carpeting, and upholstered furniture.

Our homes also contain potentially harmful plastics in many forms. One example is the polyurethane foam in furniture, which can release toxic fumes if it catches fire.

Many household paints, varnishes, adhesives, and paint removers are synthesized from petrochemicals and can release strong vapors into the air. Even when dry, they may continue to seep chemicals into a room for some time. It is healthier—and more environmentally friendly—to use water-based paints, which contain fewer harmful chemicals.

Perhaps the area over which you have most control is your choice of household cleaning products. You can improve your indoor environment by selecting nontoxic,

Safety measures in the home
Taking some basic safety precautions around your home can help to prevent a serious accident or an injury.

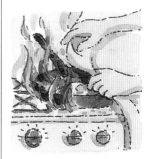

FIRE BLANKET
Keep an old wool blanket near the stove for smothering a kitchen fire instantly.

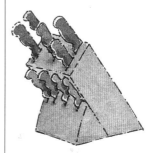

KNIFE SAFETY
Store kitchen knives out of reach of young children, ideally in a knife block.

MAKE YOUR OWN BEESWAX FURNITURE POLISH

Aerosol polishes create instant shine and make it easy to pick up dust, but they do not fill in scratches and feed the wood as wax polishes do; they can also cause surfaces to become too slippery. Continuous use can result in a milky finish, which can be removed only by stripping and refinishing the furniture. It is not necessary to always use a hard polish: wiping furniture with a damp soft cloth is often sufficient.

Beeswax is a natural furniture polish that both cleans and preserves wood, leaving a pleasant, nontoxic aroma. You can buy it or use the following recipe to make your own. For the polish you will need 55 g (2 oz) of beeswax, 140 ml (5 fl oz) of turpentine, 2 tablespoons of linseed oil, and 2 tablespoons of cedar oil.

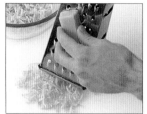

1 *Grate the beeswax and place it in a heatproof bowl.*

Stir all other ingredients into the beeswax.

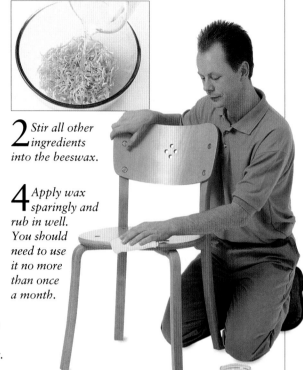

4 *Apply wax sparingly and rub in well. You should need to use it no more than once a month.*

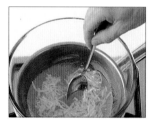

3 *Set the bowl over simmering water to melt the wax, then cool it. Take care not to breathe the vapor.*

biodegradable products, which are usually made from natural substances. A few examples are beeswax furniture polish (see above), soap made with vegetable oils and cocoa butter, dishwashing liquid and laundry detergents made with coconut oil, and laundry brighteners made with papaya enzyme. You can also find mineral deodorizers for carpets, chlorine-free mildew removers, and sink and tile cleaners that contain no abrasives or hazardous solvents.

HYGIENE

A number of health problems result from poor cleaning and storage practices in the home. The kitchen is where there is the highest risk of contamination, primarily from molds and bacteria. Germs breed on the porous surfaces of cabinets, countertops, and cutting boards. It's important to keep these surfaces clean and dry, using nontoxic products. (Recent research on antibacterial agents indicates that they are not the best choice for keeping these surfaces clean.)

When preparing food, always clean the board and knife after cutting up raw meat, poultry, or fish. Their surfaces may contain salmonella or other bacteria, which are normally destroyed by thorough cooking.

However, through careless hygiene you can inadvertently transfer them to fruits or vegetables that will be eaten raw and subsequently get very sick.

Another source of contamination is the insufficient washing of fruits and vegetables. As noted on pages 48 and 50, pesticides are widely used in farming, except in the growing of organic produce. Careful washing is essential. You can also buy products created especially for removing these residues.

Good hygiene is important in bathrooms as well. Many have inadequate ventilation, resulting in warm, damp conditions that are ideal for development of mildew and other molds. Occasional use of a mildew remover may be necessary, but it should be used sparingly and the bathroom should be well ventilated by opening the window or turning on the ventilator fan. If there is a window, opening it regularly to allow fresh air and sunlight in will limit mold growth.

Showerheads and basin and bathtub drains can easily clog and become breeding grounds for germs; they need regular cleaning. Use a plumber's snake to remove hair and pour a foaming solution of baking soda and vinegar down the drain once a month to prevent buildup of residues.

SPECIAL SAFETY NEEDS

People who are less able to care for themselves—young children and the elderly, for example—are most at risk from household hazards. Special precautions are necessary to ensure their safety.

Making a home safe for people who are especially vulnerable to its potential hazards—small children, elderly relations or friends, and the infirm or disabled—need not involve great expense or major structural work. In many cases it may be just a matter of making some very simple adjustments.

A SAFE HOME FOR CHILDREN

As most parents of young children know, the home can be a minefield of obstacles and accidents waiting to happen. An alarming number of accidents involving children occur in the home each year. These commonly involve suffocation, scalds and other burns, poisoning, and falls. Many of these injuries might be avoided with more careful attention to detail and planning.

Open staircases and windows are perhaps the most potentially dangerous areas of the home. Children love climbing on things and running up and down stairs. Older children may slide down banisters, while younger ones may use the horizontal rails as climbing frames. If the balusters are too far apart, a child's head could get stuck between them; make sure that the spaces between uprights are too narrow for this to happen. A stair safety gate can be installed inexpensively to

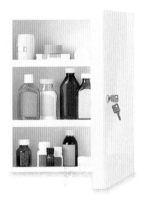

MEDICINE SAFETY
All medicines and household cleaners should be kept in well-labeled containers in cabinets with locks or childproof latches.

KEEPING CHILDREN SAFE

Accidents in the home are the most common cause of injury among young children; it is essential to be on guard all the time. Safety gadgets, which are easy to put in place, will help keep your children out of harm's way.

▶ *Keep all gas and wood fires guarded, preferably with a screen that attaches securely to the wall or fireplace.*

▶ *Unplug all electrical appliances when not in use and cover all the exposed sockets.*

▶ *Make sure you do not have any poisonous plants in the house or garden; toddlers are inclined to put everything in their mouths.*

▶ *Never leave hot drinks or saucepans containing hot liquids within a child's reach. All saucepan handles should face inward on the stove, and hot beverages should be set on a high table or counter.*

▶ *Never leave a child unsupervised in a bathtub or wading pool or near a garden pond.*

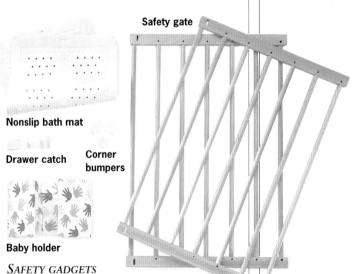

Safety gate

Nonslip bath mat

Drawer catch   **Corner bumpers**

Baby holder

SAFETY GADGETS
Drawer and cabinet catches keep little fingers out of danger; special bumpers cover sharp table corners; and baby holders keep a baby secure on his or her side or back. These accessories are quick to install in your home.

BEDROOM COMFORT

Children are particularly sensitive to chemical toxins and sleep more than adults do, so it is vital to make their bedrooms safe. Follow these simple steps to create an environment conducive to a healthy and good night's sleep.

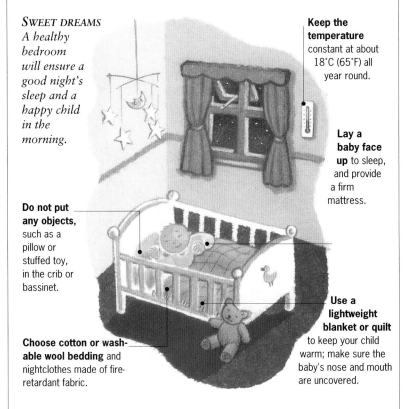

SWEET DREAMS
A healthy bedroom will ensure a good night's sleep and a happy child in the morning.

Keep the temperature constant at about 18°C (65°F) all year round.

Lay a baby face up to sleep, and provide a firm mattress.

Do not put any objects, such as a pillow or stuffed toy, in the crib or bassinet.

Choose cotton or washable wool bedding and nightclothes made of fire-retardant fabric.

Use a lightweight blanket or quilt to keep your child warm; make sure the baby's nose and mouth are uncovered.

It is advisable never to leave children unsupervised in a room with a fire, even if the fireplace is screened; a child might pull the screen over. It is wise also to keep children well away from bonfires and barbecue grills, and never use any flammable liquids to start a fire. Make sure also that children are supervised while watching fireworks.

Small children often have a habit of putting their fingers into power sockets, while older children may attempt to plug in electrical appliances. Unused sockets should have safety covers. Furniture should be placed in front of lamp and appliance cords that are plugged in or cords taped to the wall. Allow children to use the television and VCR only under adult supervision, and fit a video recorder with a cover that prevents them from fiddling with the buttons and the tape-loading mechanism.

Keep medicines and household chemicals well away from children. A high cabinet not reachable by climbing is the best place to store them. A good alternative is to put safety catches on all cabinets in the kitchen and bathroom. Never put household cleaners into soft-drink bottles, where they might look like tempting treats. And keep your vitamins and minerals in childproof bottles. Every year hundreds of children are poisoned by swallowing megadoses.

If you have outdoor play equipment, check it regularly to be sure it is in good repair. Wading pools should be covered

keep toddlers from getting near a stairway, but it is advisable not to let older children play near or on a staircase at all.

Windows pose another threat. To prevent accidents, fit horizontal safety bars in the lower part of window openings and keep the keys in a safe place nearby to allow escape in case of fire. Alternatively, place screws in the window frame to keep the window from opening fully. This will allow air in but will prevent a child from falling out. Ideally, doors and windows should be fitted with safety glass to make them difficult to break accidentally. Also, don't put a bunk bed near a window if you can avoid it.

Fit covers over all radiators to prevent burns from contact with hot metal. If you use a space heater, choose a model with ceramic heating discs (rather than heating coils), shielded fan blades, and an automatic shut-off system in case the unit overheats or tips over. The casing of such heaters stays cool to the touch and cannot burn the skin.

PREVENTING CRIB DEATH

Research by two Americans, Joseph Hattersley and Lendon Smith, published in 1998 in the *International Journal of Alternative and Complementary Medicine*, suggested that the bedding used in a baby's bassinet or crib may be a factor in sudden infant death syndrome (SID), or crib death. A common household fungus, *Scopularis brevicaulis*, consumes the plastic used in some baby mattresses, and the process releases phosphine, arsine, and stibine, which are odorless, highly poisonous gases. More research needs to be done, however.

The annual number of crib deaths has gone down since parents were advised to put infants to bed on their backs.

when not in use. Swimming pools should be enclosed with a fence and a lockable gate (this is the law in many places). Never allow children to swim unsupervised.

Children's rooms

Babies and young children are particularly sensitive to chemical toxins because of the immaturity of their immune and lung systems and their high metabolic rate. A large percentage of their time is spent indoors, making them more vulnerable to the home environment. Their smaller body size and faster breathing rate means that air quality and temperature easily affect their well-being, especially in their bedroom.

The effect of chemicals in baby mattresses remains a controversial subject. However, recent evidence has suggested that some chemicals might play a role in infant crib death (see opposite page). Babies may also suffer other problems related to allergic reactions caused by dust mites, chemical fabric treatments, whiteners, and softeners. It is better to use bedding and clothing made of natural fibers, such as cotton, rather than synthetics. Sheets free of formaldehyde and whitened by environmentally safe hydrogen peroxide are readily available, as are unbleached cotton and wool blankets. Dust-mite-proof mattress and pillow covers are also a good investment.

A SAFE HOME FOR THE ELDERLY

The elderly spend a great deal of time indoors, especially if they are infirm or unwell, so it is important that their homes present as few hazards as possible.

Interiors should be well lit—with each room fitted with a central light turned on by a wall switch, as well as reading and work lights. Light switches should be accessible and easy to manipulate, cords should be tucked under rugs and behind furniture, and there should be a night-light to reduce the danger of tripping in the dark.

Harmful cleaning products

Most cleaning products found in the home contain chemicals that can cause dry and itchy skin conditions, and the fumes they emit can irritate the throat and lungs. It is much better to use cleaning products that are formulated to be safe for the environment. These are widely available today from many catalogs and stores.

MINIMIZING BATHROOM HAZARDS

The bathroom is a potential site of serious accidents for everyone, but young children and the frail elderly are the most at risk. The damp atmosphere in bathrooms can attract bacteria and mold, as well as cause surfaces to become very slippery. By making a few small adjustments, most accidents can be avoided.

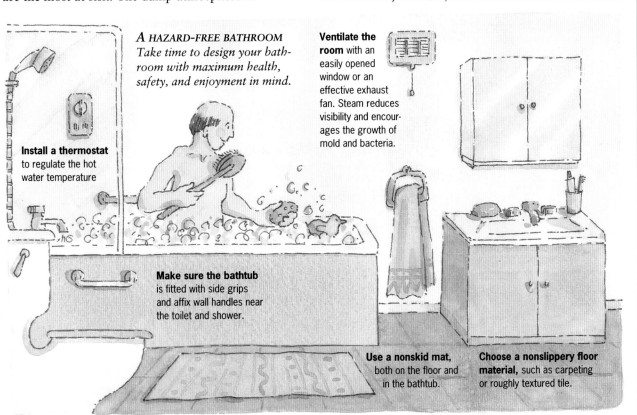

A HAZARD-FREE BATHROOM
Take time to design your bathroom with maximum health, safety, and enjoyment in mind.

Ventilate the room with an easily opened window or an effective exhaust fan. Steam reduces visibility and encourages the growth of mold and bacteria.

Install a thermostat to regulate the hot water temperature

Make sure the bathtub is fitted with side grips and affix wall handles near the toilet and shower.

Use a nonskid mat, both on the floor and in the bathtub.

Choose a nonslippery floor material, such as carpeting or roughly textured tile.

FEELING SAFER IN THE HOME

Some simple gadgets and home improvements can make a big difference in how safe elderly people feel in their homes. An older person who can maintain current levels of independence with improved comfort and safety will continue to enjoy his or her own living space for a longer period.

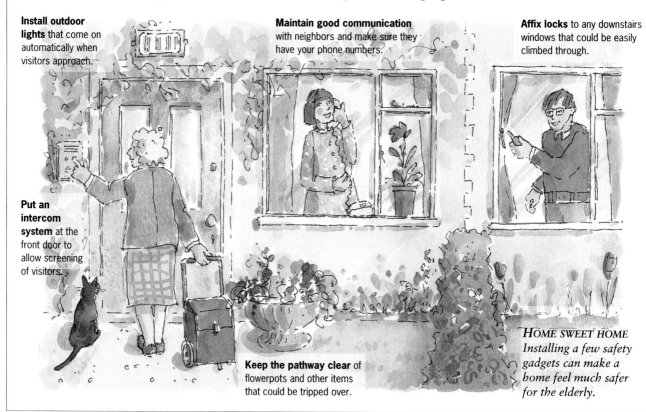

Install outdoor lights that come on automatically when visitors approach.

Maintain good communication with neighbors and make sure they have your phone numbers.

Affix locks to any downstairs windows that could be easily climbed through.

Put an intercom system at the front door to allow screening of visitors.

Keep the pathway clear of flowerpots and other items that could be tripped over.

HOME SWEET HOME Installing a few safety gadgets can make a home feel much safer for the elderly.

It is important that an elderly person's home be free from unnecessary clutter, too; items that block doorways and floor spaces could cause injury. Carpets should be well fitted, and scatter rugs should have a pad that prevents them from slipping; the edges of scatter rugs can also be taped to the floor to prevent tripping over them.

Although some people lose at least part of their hearing when they age, many older people become very sensitive to noise, especially at night. Loud music, television sets, and general chatter can cause distress, so make sure that rooms are carpeted and otherwise made as soundproof as possible.

To prevent tripping over trailing cords from lamps or electrical appliances, you can buy a gadget that keeps a cord coiled inside. Keep plugs and wiring in good condition and never overload power sockets or extension cords, which can become overheated. Fit smoke alarms throughout the house. (For people who are hearing impaired, there are types that flash lights when triggered.) Keep air vents unblocked to ensure good ventilation and have gas appliances properly installed and well maintained. Also, clearly label medicine and pill bottles, especially if several different pills need to be taken. Color coding can be helpful for keeping them sorted out.

As people grow older, they become less able to cope with fluctuations in temperature. Home insulation, windows that are double-glazed, and insulated draperies and shades help keep the indoor temperature steadier. Because many elderly people live on limited budgets, heat should not be wasted. It is better for the heating to be controlled automatically so that a constant temperature is maintained all year round.

For security, install a light outside every entrance door and fit the door with a chain and spy hole. The telephone and doorbell should be easily heard in all areas of the house, and if possible, there should be more than one telephone so there is a better chance of getting help in an emergency.

SPACE, LIGHT, AND COLOR

When space, light, and color work harmoniously within your home, the result can be a truly healthful, pleasurable, and comfortable environment.

Well-planned space, adequate and glare-free lighting, and pleasing color schemes in a home can bring benefits for both physical and mental health. Most people are aware of the stress that arises from lack of personal space, the effect of color in reinforcing particular moods, and the distraction of clutter, which can interfere with the ability to think clearly and act freely. However, these factors can also affect physical health. Too many objects and pieces of furniture can encourage the growth of allergy triggers, such as dust mites and mold, while inadequate lighting can strain your eyes or cause accidents.

CLEARING THE CLUTTER
Everyone should examine the extent to which space at home is overwhelmed by unnecessary items. Many people accumulate objects that they don't need but may be reluctant to throw out because the items carry sentimental value. But clutter collects dust and can also develop mold, and these can cause health problems, including allergies and breathing difficulties. Some types of clutter—magazines and newspapers, for example—can also be a fire hazard, igniting during hot weather from spontaneous combustion. Though not necessarily a hazard, a musty smell can also accumulate around clutter if a home is not aired regularly. Fresh air should flow regularly through the house.

The dust that settles into upholstered furnishings, curtains, bedding, and carpets and lurks around ornaments and pictures can harbor microscopic dust mites. They thrive in warm, damp conditions, feeding off human skin scales. During its three-month life span, one dust mite lays 20 to 40 eggs and produces up to 2,000 droppings that can trigger respiratory problems and certain types of skin conditions. The average indoor temperature in homes today—68°F—is the perfect temperature for house dust mites to proliferate. This may be one reason that incidences of allergy have increased in recent years. To combat dust mites, regularly air and clean your bedding, carpets, and curtains. Because vacuuming tends to recirculate dust mites into the air, it's best to use special bags and a filter that trap them.

MAKING THE MOST OF SPACE
You may be able to improve your existing storage space with a few adaptations, such as adding extra shelves, drawers, or bins to the inside of cabinets or closets. If you do

---

REDUCING DUST IN YOUR HOME

Even if you or your family members do not suffer from dust-related allergies, it is still beneficial to minimize the amount of dust-collecting on surfaces in your home.

▶ *Choose enclosed, glass-fronted bookcases rather than open ones. Books are difficult to keep dust-free on open shelves and can also harbor molds.*

▶ *Increase the ventilation in your home and do not overheat it. Dust mites thrive in calm, warm, and humid environments.*

▶ *Vacuum regularly to remove dust from upholstered furniture and carpets and have them steam-cleaned at least once a year.*

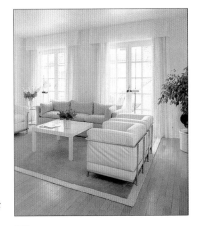

WOOD FLOORS
Wood floors are a good choice for keeping dust mites at bay. Even area rugs can harbor them, so rugs should be cleaned regularly.

CREATIVE STORAGE IDEAS

If you have cleared as much clutter as possible from your home but find that possessions are still overflowing the available storage space, consider other places and ways for housing accessories, bathroom products, magazines, and bedding. Many storage products can double as decorative features in a room.

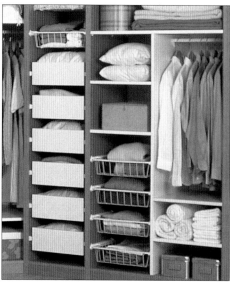

WARDROBE STORAGE
Maximize space with a built-in closet that includes adjustable shelves, drawers, closet rods, pull-out wire baskets, and shoe racks.

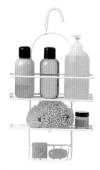

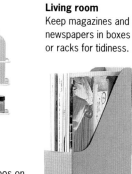

Living room
Keep magazines and newspapers in boxes or racks for tidiness.

Bathroom
Keep soaps and shampoos on a shower rack for easy access and storage.

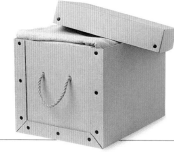

Bedroom
Store bedding and seasonal clothing in boxes at the back of the closet or under the bed.

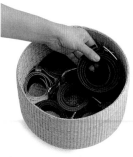

ACCESSORY STORAGE
You can store belts in a basket or round box, preferably one with a lid to keep out dust.

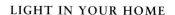

not have a spare room, cellar, or attic, you will have to be imaginative about increasing storage in your living space. Shelving can be fitted to most walls if the supports are attached to studs. In the kitchen the ceiling can be adapted to provide hanging space for saucepans and utensils, while in the bedroom, items can be stored conveniently in drawers or boxes under the bed.

Ample storage is essential in the kitchen. Installing tiered shelving in top cupboards makes better use of space, and putting a carousel in a cabinet improves accessibility to difficult corners. If you are creating new storage areas, design these in a way that allows you to reach things easily. When you are building storage space for children or the elderly, you should locate doorknobs and shelves within easy reach.

LIGHT IN YOUR HOME

Light influences your psychological health; using it effectively is a vital part of making the home comfortable and healthy. Well-lit areas enable you to work and read without straining your eyes, whereas softly lit areas foster rest and relaxation. Natural light contains electromagnetic energy, which is essential to life and affects many physiological and psychological processes in the body. Among other things it influences the pituitary and pineal glands, both master glands of the endocrine system, which control the release in the body of hormones that are closely linked to moods and emotions. If you are one of the many people today who spend long periods indoors under artificial light, it is essential to find ways to let as much natural light as possible into your living and working spaces and, if this isn't possible, to use lighting that simulates daylight.

Incandescent lights (ordinary household lightbulbs) give off more red light than normal daylight. In fact, most incandescent lights produce more infrared heat than light. It is possible to buy clear, regular white, soft white, or tinted bulbs, each of which produces a different effect. "Daylight" bulbs, which are more balanced in their spectrum, are often used by artists because they

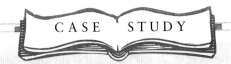

CASE STUDY

A Depressed Woman

Arthritis at any age, but especially in an older person, can be very debilitating. The intense pain in joints can make movement difficult, even impossible, and can cause the sufferer to become housebound and isolated. Social activities, regular exercise, and a healthy diet are often sacrificed because of the difficulty of leaving the house, and depression can eventually set in.

Ellen is 72 and lives alone in a small town. She has suffered from osteoarthritis in her knees and hips for several years, but the pain has recently become much worse. Ellen has always been very independent, yet for the past few weeks she has been housebound and has not even attended her regular church service or the lunch club in which she has long been an active member.

Spending most of her time indoors on her own has made her depressed and lonely; on some days she does not even open the shades or get up to cook. Ellen's doctor did give her some drugs for the arthritis pain and advised a healthy diet, moderate exercise, and plenty of fresh air, but somehow this advice seems easier said than followed.

WHAT SHOULD ELLEN DO?

Ellen must first do all she can to improve her arthritis. She should eat plenty of fresh fruits and vegetables, which are high in the antioxidant vitamins A, C, and E; vitamin C especially may lower the risk of cartilage loss and inhibit progression of the disease. She might inquire if her town offers bus service to the market for senior citizens.

Ellen should also make sure that her indoor environment is healthy by clearing out any clutter and opening the windows every day to admit fresh air and light. Ellen should also try to make herself walk to the end of the street every day to buy a paper because the exercise will help, and she should resume her social activities as soon as possible.

Action Plan

EMOTIONS
Recognize the importance of regular social interaction and ask a friend or two to share driving to church and social events.

LIFESTYLE
Make sure that each day has a structure, with time allotted for meal preparation and gentle exercise. Keep the house clean and well aired and get outdoors as often as possible.

DIET
Eat three regular meals a day and include at least five servings of fruits and vegetables.

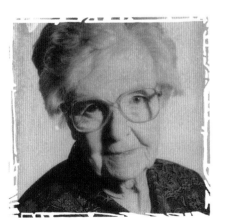

DIET
Not eating properly can exacerbate existing problems and cause more severe symptoms to develop.

EMOTIONS
Not being able to continue a regular social life in old age can have an adverse effect on physical and mental health.

LIFESTYLE
Depression is a vicious circle. Being indoors all the time increases lethargy because a lack of fresh air and light can make a person morose.

HOW THINGS TURNED OUT FOR ELLEN

Ellen asked a friend to help her clear some clutter that was blocking access to windows in her house so she couldn't let in air and light. They placed a chair by a window where Ellen can sit and read. She walks every day and gets a weekly ride to the supermarket, which is improving her diet. She is feeling less depressed and has become more socially active, but she still suffers pain. In the longer term she is considering moving to a retirement home.

CHOOSING LIGHT FOR YOUR HOME

The quality of lighting in your home is of great importance. It can affect your moods, energy levels, and concentration and make a room homey or not. When choosing electric lights for your home, it is recommended that you use a variety of different types, depending on the needs of each individual space.

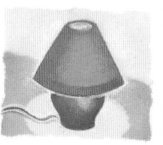

COLORED LIGHTING
Low-level lighting using a tinted or colored bulb or shade provides a restful mood but is not good for tasks.

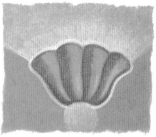

UP LIGHTING
An alternative to harsh over-head lighting, up lighting brightens spots in a room and creates a softer atmosphere.

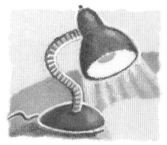

SPOT LIGHTING
Suited to close-up work, such as reading, cooking, sewing, and needlework, spot lighting prevents eyestrain.

provide a truer, more natural light than clear or regular lightbulbs. Pink bulbs give off a soft, warm light.

Most fluorescent tubes emit more ultraviolet light, which can give all the colors in a room a bluish tinge. These lights also pulse, and though you may not notice at first, older tubes often hum and flicker. Together with fluorescent glare and UV emissions, this type of lighting can cause eyestrain, headaches, and irritability. Some newer fluorescent tubes are more efficient, healthier, and longer lasting than the older type and are available in warmer hues. Also, the flicker is 10 times faster, so it is invisible to the eye, and the hum is so high pitched, it is inaudible. Compact fluorescent bulbs are now available that can be used in place of incandescent bulbs. An advantage of fluorescent lighting is that it emits less heat than other types and thus attracts less dust. It also uses much less electricity and therefore saves money and produces less pollution.

Tungsten-halogen bulbs give off a bright light that is very close to daylight in quality. They are powerful and effective for general illumination. Low-voltage ones are more energy efficient and are ideal for spot lighting and accents. Tungsten-halogen bulbs are expensive, but they have a very long life.

COLORS IN YOUR HOME

Lighting is not the only way in which to alter mood. The colors you choose for a room can also affect your psychological state.

When deciding on an interior color scheme, you need to take several things into account—the architectural style, the existing furnishings, the availability of natural light and the hours during which it enters the room, the atmosphere you wish to create, and the personal tastes and preferences of those who will be using the room.

Being surrounded by a certain color can have a profound effect on the human psyche, although the effect is often a subtle and unconscious one. If you understand the emotional qualities of colors, you can use this knowledge to good advantage when selecting hues for different rooms in the house (see chart, opposite page).

*CREATING MOOD
WITH LIGHT
The type of lighting chosen for a room will affect its overall feel. Soft lighting creates a homey, comfortable atmosphere, ideal for rest and relaxation. This living room has a variety of subtle artificial light sources, as well as natural light from the large windows.*

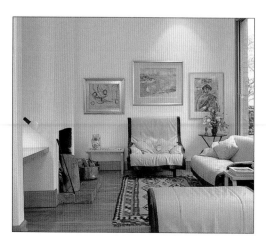

Warm colors, such as red and yellow, can create a stimulating and happy atmosphere and thus are good choices for a family room, kitchen, or dining room, where social interaction is desired. Cool colors, such as blues and purples, are more peaceful and calming, making them ideal for use in a bedroom or any other room where time is spent resting and relaxing. Neutral colors, like white, cream, and beige, also have a calming effect.

Not only a particular color itself but the intensity of it—whether it is a deep shade or light tint—and how much gray has been added to tone it down will determine its psychological effect. Lighter, grayed tones are easier to live with than intense, bright ones, which can be too stimulating if used on walls. Light colors also reflect more light, making a room seem larger and brighter, which can also lighten the mood.

THE EMOTIONAL QUALITIES OF COLOR

Color has a profound effect on our emotions, so much so that it is often used in therapy. For example, some hospitals use red blankets because red promotes healing and energy. And institutions are often painted a calming white or pale green. The table below shows the qualities of different colors and what rooms they are best for. Of course, this is only a guide, and there is no reason why you should not break the rules if you have different color preferences.

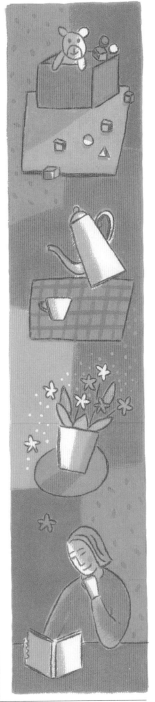

COLOR	EFFECTS	BEST SITUATION
Red (crimson, scarlet, wine)	Stimulates the muscles; raises the pulse and blood pressure.	Use in areas in which you are active or wish to create movement, such as the hall, stairs, kitchen, or family room.
Pink (deep rose, salmon, pale pink)	Gently stimulates; relaxes the muscles; is emotionally supportive and uplifting.	Use in areas in which you wish to give emotional support, such as children's rooms, rooms for the elderly, bedrooms.
Orange (peach, apricot, terra-cotta)	Has releasing and opening action on body systems, especially reproductive organs; stimulates appetite; uplifts the mind.	Use in the kitchen and dining room and other areas where you wish to create a warm atmosphere and encourage social interchange.
Yellow (gold, cream)	Strengthens nerves; stimulates liver and gallbladder; is mentally stimulating.	Creates a happy or vibrant atmosphere; good for studies and rooms with low natural light; has good light-reflecting properties.
Green (fresh bright and light tones, emerald)	Relaxes the muscles around the heart and lungs; is good for the digestion; eliminates toxins; balances emotions; is calming, relaxing, and balancing; helps connect with natural rhythms; aids recuperation after illness.	As a neutral, balancing color, it can be introduced in the form of plants into all rooms.
Blue (royal, sky and other light hues)	Is sedating; depresses appetite; is anti-inflammatory; is soothing to the throat and lungs. Creates a peaceful and cool atmosphere.	Use in moderation along with some warm colors for balance; is good in a bedroom or bathroom.
Purple (lavender, orchid, mauve)	Balances the mind and the psyche; feeds central nervous system and spine; is cleansing to the blood; has transformative and inspirational qualities.	Use in areas where you wish to be creative or spiritual; creates an air of luxury and richness.
Brown (tan, beige, mushroom)	Has an earthy grounding quality; aids practicality; provides protection; use to create a neutral backdrop to highlight other colors.	Is best used in natural materials, such as wood, natural fabrics, and ceramics.

FENG SHUI

Devotees of feng shui believe that practicing this ancient approach to interior design in your home can do much to improve your health and happiness and that of your family.

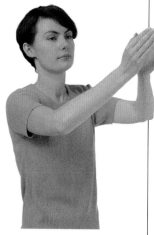

HAND CLAPPING
Feng shui practitioners carry out various forms of space clearing, such as clapping loudly in corners and near the walls of a building to disperse stagnant energy.

Feng shui (pronounced feng shway) is an ancient Chinese art that seeks to arrange an environment to promote optimum health and well-being. It is based partly on common sense and partly on interpretation of the cosmological forces of the universe. Its underlying premise is that everything in your environment, down to the smallest detail, can affect you physically, emotionally, and spiritually.

A feng shui consultant is often brought in when a family, person, or business is suffering from a physical, emotional, or mental trauma that has no obvious cause. It may be that they have experienced a run of bad luck, a bout of serious illness, or an emotional problem that seems to have coincided with moving into a new home or changing to a new place of business.

The aim of feng shui is to maximize the flow of chi, or life force energy. This energy is constantly on the move, flowing in gently sweeping curves through the landscape, your home, and your body. In order for harmony to reign inside your home, chi must flow freely from the outside through the interior and back out again. Therefore, the size and placement of entrance doors and interior objects are important. Wherever chi is blocked, a feng shui practitioner will try to enhance its energy with such devices as mirrors, wind chimes, or mobiles, positioning them carefully for the best effect.

SPACE CLEARING

If strong emotions have been generated in a room, feng shui practitioners counsel that it is wise to clear the room of any negative energy. They believe that such negativity tends to linger in the furniture and appurtenances and is even absorbed by the walls.

One of the first things to do when clearing space is to give your home a thorough spring cleaning. Stagnant energy, like dust,

PREVENTING BLOCKED CHI

There are several places within a home where the natural flow of chi can become blocked. Once these areas are cleaned out or altered, it is often striking how fresh a house feels and how much the atmosphere is improved. The following areas are common places for chi to become stagnant or trapped.

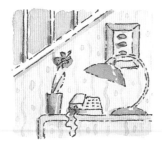

UNDER STAIRS
Keep well lit and painted in a light color. Clear clutter and, if possible, add a window in the area to let in natural light.

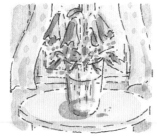

SELDOM USED ROOMS
Open a window to allow fresh air to circulate and add plants or fresh flowers to enliven the atmosphere.

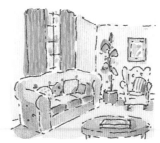

LARGE FURNITURE
Place large items of furniture in a room that is spacious enough to allow chi to flow easily around them.

EIGHT DIRECTIONS

Many feng shui practitioners believe that a distinctive form of energy characterizes a room, home, or landscape according to its orientation. A room on the east side, for example, will encourage self-confidence, optimism, and activity.

COMPASS DIRECTIONS AND CHI
Each point of the compass is associated with a different kind of chi. If possible, rooms should correspond to the chi that best suits their function.

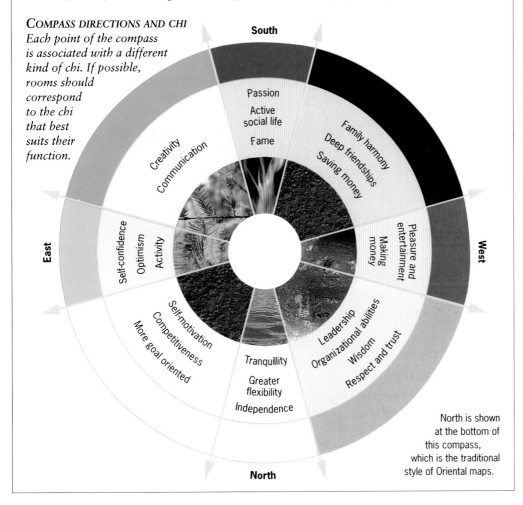

North is shown at the bottom of this compass, which is the traditional style of Oriental maps.

South

Passion
Active social life
Fame

Family harmony
Deep friendships
Saving money

Creativity
Communication

Pleasure and entertainment

East

Self-confidence
Optimism
Activity

Making money

West

Self-motivation
Competitiveness
More goal oriented

Leadership
Organizational abilities
Wisdom
Respect and trust

Tranquillity
Greater flexibility
Independence

North

collects in corners or unused places, and cleaning will dislodge and disperse it. Try also to repair any items that are broken or recycle anything that is beyond repair; otherwise, they simply represent redundant clutter. Similarly, tackle any outstanding tasks, such as letter writing or mending, that you have been putting off. Seeing a coat with a missing button or a broken clock when you enter a room will sap your energy subconsciously. Most people find it easier to think and go forward with their lives if their homes are clean and tidy.

PRINCIPLE OF EIGHT DIRECTIONS

One important aspect of feng shui is the principle holding that each of the eight points on the compass is associated with a different kind of chi. Each compass direc-

tion encompasses both yin and yang (passive and active energies) and is linked also to the following: one of the five elements (metal, earth, water, fire, and air); a symbol of the natural world; a family member; a number in Oriental astrology that determines individual characteristics according to date of birth; a color; a time of day; and a season. Together these create a detailed picture of the type of chi that will affect anything placed in that section of a house or piece of land, including the general siting of a house, the location of individual rooms, and the position of furniture and other objects within the rooms.

The next seven pages provide some rudimentary guidelines on how to apply the principles of feng shui in order to encourage the most advantageous flow of chi in each room of your home.

Yin and yang
One of the fundamental principles of feng shui is that everything in the world can be seen in terms of two kinds of energy—passive and active, or yin and yang. Yang is the positive force and is characteristically aggressive, dynamic, stimulating, and energetic. Yin, the counterbalancing negative force, is characteristically peaceful, creative, sensitive, and calm.

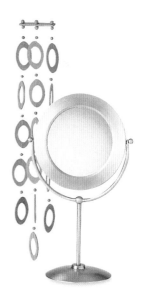

ENHANCING ENERGY
Mirrors and wind chimes are particularly effective at stimulating and dispersing chi. Mirrors reflect chi in several directions to spread it around, and wind chimes cleanse energy in areas prone to stagnation.

105

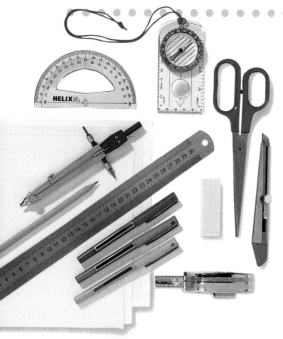

FLOOR PLAN

The practice of some forms of feng shui relies on knowing the compass directions of your home and where each room lies within that framework. An important first step, therefore, is to draw a floor plan showing the size and orientation of the rooms.

ESSENTIAL EQUIPMENT
To create a feng shui floor plan, you will need colored pens, a pencil, ruler, tape measure, sheet of graph paper for each floor of the house, some tracing paper, cardboard, and a compass.

Many practitioners of feng shui believe that the eight directions spanning outward from the center point of a building have specific energies. In order to make use of these different energies in your home, you first need to draw a detailed floor plan (see below) and align it with a grid of the eight directions (see page 105). If the house has more than one floor, a separate plan should be drafted for each floor.

Once you have finished the floor plan, you can find the precise compass direction of each room by positioning the eight-directions grid over the plan. With this knowledge you will be able to assess the type of chi in each room so that you can match or adapt the room's activities to suit its supportive chi. This concept can be applied to any space that you occupy, whether it's a house, apartment, or office.

MAKING YOUR OWN FLOOR PLAN

To create a floor plan of your home that can act as a feng shui guide, you will need a compass (the one shown here is conveniently attached to a ruler). Compasses can become unbalanced by things made of iron or by electronic items like a television. Take readings from various places until the reading is consistent in several parts of a room.

1 *On graph paper, draw the outline of each floor of your home to scale—for example, three squares equal one foot. Then measure the dimensions of each room and corridor and draw them into the outline. Sketch in all windows and doorways and also large movable pieces of furniture.*

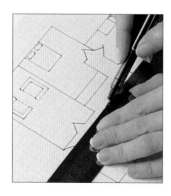

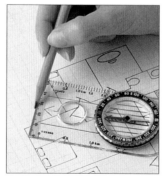

3 *Line up the floor plan with your home, using your front door as a guide. Then locate the direction of magnetic north in relation to your home, using the compass. Lay the compass on the floor plan and draw a straight line from the center point of your home to an outside wall in the direction of magnetic north.*

2 *Find the center point of your floor plan. If it is roughly rectangular or square, draw lines from each corner to the opposite corner. The point where they cross is the center. If it is an uneven shape, paste the plan onto cardboard, cut it out, and balance it on the tip of a pencil. The point where the plan balances is the center.*

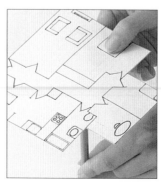

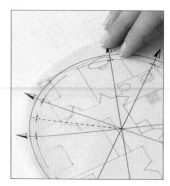

4 *Trace the eight directions diagram from page 105 onto a sheet of transparent paper. Place the tracing on top of your floor plan, aligning the center points and the lines showing magnetic north. You will now be able to assess which energies influence the individual rooms.*

LIVING ROOM

The living room in many homes has to fulfill a variety of functions. It may be the principal area for everyday relaxation, as well as a welcoming environment for guests and a suitable place for celebrating important occasions.

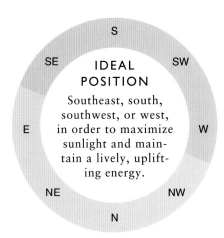

IDEAL POSITION
Southeast, south, southwest, or west, in order to maximize sunlight and maintain a lively, uplifting energy.

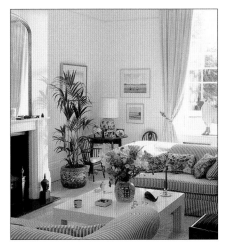

THE IDEAL SPACE
This living room embodies many feng shui principles. The pale colors of the walls, the positioning of the sofas, the wooden floor, and the fireplace combine to create a harmonious atmosphere.

Feng shui practitioners believe that the best position for a living room is in the southeast, south, southwest, or west area of your home, where it will receive a good amount of sunlight during the day, which stimulates the flow of chi for a lively atmosphere.

If entertaining is an important aspect of your lifestyle, the south is a good choice because it is lively and bright and so is especially favorable for holding social events. If a cosy, calm atmosphere is more important, then the southwest or west are better positions because they have a romantic character.

Feng shui consultants often recommend bare floors in living rooms to maintain a harmonious flow of chi, with a pure wool rug added for comfort. To encourage a relaxing atmosphere, patterned wallpaper is recommended rather than plain painted walls; green and white vertical stripes are uplifting. If your room feels stagnant, try adding a water feature in the form of an aquarium, which will encourage a favorable flow of chi.

One of the most important features of a living room is the fireplace, which brings a comfortable and warming aspect to the home during winter. Practitioners believe that it can also increase excitement, passion, spontaneity, and brightness. It is therefore important to position a fireplace where it will be most beneficial. The northern side of the building, where the energy is colder and more yin, better complements the warmer, yang fire energy. To reflect more chi into a room, place a mirror above the fireplace. If it is not possible to have a fireplace in your home, various objects can have a similar effect. For example, candles, bright lights, and furnishings in yang colors, like bright yellow, orange, and red, can be effective.

Plants add life and absorb the negative emissions of a television set. Tall palms are uplifting in large rooms, whereas round-leaved bushy plants are more appropriate in small rooms.

ENCOURAGING CHI
The main goal of a living room is to promote comfort and relaxation. Feng shui consultants recommend yin colors of pale purple, green, blue, and cream.

The position of chairs and sofas has a major impact on the atmosphere of a living room. To promote family harmony, place the sofa in the northwest facing southeast, with two chairs in front, opposite each other— one in the northeast facing southwest and the other in southwest facing northeast; then put one chair in the southeast facing northwest to complete the social circle.

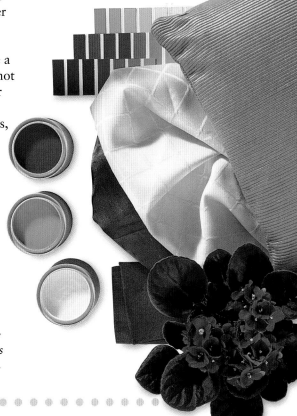

DINING ROOM

The function of a dining room can vary dramatically. A formal dinner for special guests, for instance, is very different from a casual family gathering. In each case, however, good communication is the central aim.

Whole-grain bread is more yang than white bread.

Sparkling glasses act with the cutlery to bounce chi around the table.

Reflective plates and cutlery move chi around the table.

Red accessories, in the form of candles, roses, and napkins, add dynamic elements.

Feng shui recognizes the central role of food to our well-being; therefore, the dining room is of particular importance in the home. Sitting down to a meal with the family not only improves digestion but also facilitates interaction. According to feng shui, the best position for a dining room is the east, southeast, west, or northwest side of the home. East encourages liveliness and ambition, while the southeast encourages communication. West and northwest favor wisdom and contentment.

Furnishings that are easy to clean and comfortable will encourage a relaxing and convivial atmosphere. Carpets are not advised unless they are easily cleaned. Natural-colored wood is ideal because it has a neutral effect on chi and is easy to maintain. A mirror positioned to reflect the table enhances the chi of food.

Consider using fabric shades or venetian blinds as window coverings rather than curtains, which cause chi to stagnate. Candles are a good lighting option because they add fire energy, helping to produce warmth and vibrancy. Paintings of restful landscapes or festive scenes help to create a positive ambience.

SEATING YOUR GUESTS

In feng shui each position around the dining table is associated with a family member or guest who embodies the dominant chi of that location. You can use this energy to enhance both family gatherings and more formal dinner parties. Sitting

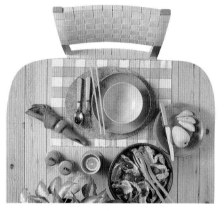

A YIN TABLE SETTING
To create a relaxed atmosphere, set a yin table, using linens of natural fiber, earthenware plates, and wood-handled cutlery, which all calm the flow of chi.

on the south side of the table facing north brings out the expressive side of people; on the north side facing south is a position of stillness and passion. Chi is playful for someone sitting on the west side facing east; sitting on the east side facing west is connected with action and ambition.

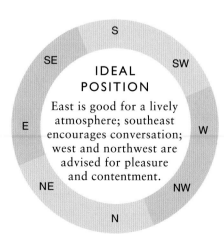

IDEAL POSITION

East is good for a lively atmosphere; southeast encourages conversation; west and northwest are advised for pleasure and contentment.

A YANG TABLE SETTING
For an exciting and stimulating effect in a table setting, use a yang approach. This includes reflective surfaces of cutlery and sparkling glassware, which spin chi around the table. Candles and touches of red add fire and passion. Strong yang foods like salmon and whole-grain bread help to complete the effect.

KITCHEN

Feng shui practitioners believe that food preparation is influenced by the surrounding chi, so choosing a favorable location is important. The positioning of the stove and sink is also crucial.

Feng shui practitioners recommend that your kitchen be located east or southeast of the center of your home because this encourages bright, uplifting energy, supportive of growth and creative activity. If possible, avoid placing the kitchen in the northeast, where the cold, piercing, and quick-changing chi is less conducive to the creation of healthy, well-balanced meals. Because kitchens combine the incompatible elements of fire and water, these must be carefully placed so that their energy is harmonized.

Try to obtain as much natural light in the kitchen as possible. Sunlight not only is uplifting but also helps

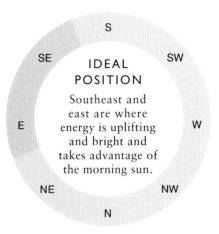

IDEAL POSITION

Southeast and east are where energy is uplifting and bright and takes advantage of the morning sun.

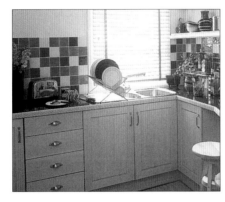

DESIGNING THE KITCHEN
Feng shui practitioners believe that wood is the ideal surface for food preparation and that cabinets, shelves, and counter-tops should have rounded corners to avoid cutting the flow of chi.

keep the kitchen dry, encouraging fresh, clean energy. Good ventilation should be a priority.

Choose cabinets with rounded edges and countertops with rounded corners to prevent cutting chi, and try not to clutter the kitchen with too many utensils and appliances, which can cause stagnation. Wood surfaces are ideal, and plants harmonize the fire and water elements. Bowls of fruit and vases of flowers promote a healthy flow of chi.

KITCHEN COLORS
Blues and greens enhance the chi favorable to the kitchen, and images of vegetables and fruits are harmonious and compatible. Cork tiles are a perfect type of yin floor.

Cooking Directions

Feng shui practitioners believe that your meals are influenced by the direction you face while cooking. East and southeast are both ideal positions. The east favors activity and practicality. The southeast encourages creativity and communication and a positive outlook. Facing north is the least propitious direction because the chi is too quiet there for the generally dynamic nature of preparing a meal. Facing west is settling; although this could be helpful for perfectionist cooks, in others it could encourage laziness.

CHOOSING THE STOVE

The stove holds an important position in feng shui because the food prepared on it contributes to the creation of life in your body. As the most important appliance in the kitchen, it should be as large as space permits. If you have a choice, feng shui favors gas stoves because electric stoves (and microwave ovens) emit radiation that can negatively affect chi.

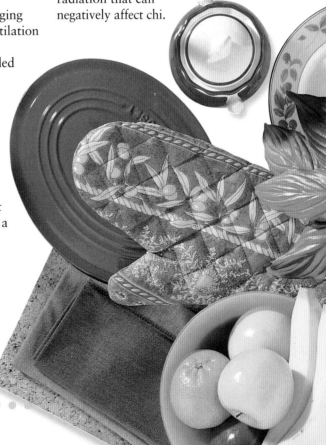

BATHROOM

Bathrooms present particular feng shui challenges. Continual dampness can lead to a heavier flow of chi and stagnation, while the draining of bathroom fixtures can flush away beneficial chi.

Colorful ceramic tiles speed the flow of chi to create a stimulating environment.

Blues and greens are ideal for accessories, such as towels, especially in the east and southeast.

Plants stimulate chi and absorb moisture.

Hard, smooth, reflective materials facilitate the flow of chi and prevent stagnation.

BATHROOM ACCESSORIES
Furniture and bric-a-brac should be kept to a minimum, and surfaces should be kept dry and clean to prevent stagnation of chi. Leafy plants make the room feel fresh and alive and absorb the humidity from showering and bathing.

The draining effect of showers, bathtubs, and toilets in bathrooms is thought to exhaust the energy in the rest of the house, so the location of a bathroom is important. Here are some points to try to observe: If possible, do not locate a bathroom near a staircase, opposite the main entrance door, or right next to the dining room or kitchen.

The most favorable position for a bathroom is in the east or southeast part of the house because the sun on this side will keep the room drier and prevent stagnation, and natural light in the morning will help stimulate chi. If your bathroom is an internal room with no window, feng shui suggests the installation of bright lights to mimic the effect of natural light.

Ventilation is also vital to the circulation of chi. You should open a window every day; if this is not possible, use the exhaust fan to aid in controlling humidity. Leafy plants will make the room feel fresher and help to maintain the flow of chi.

Ceramic tiles, a yang material, are an acceptable choice for flooring and walls because shiny surfaces help to stimulate chi. Mirrors can also be useful for encouraging energy flow, and they help make a room seem larger; however, you should avoid hanging two mirrors opposite each other because the chi will be caught up in an endless back-and-forth movement.

The toilet should be positioned well away from the bathroom door to reduce its draining effect on the rest of the house. Keep the lid closed when the toilet is not in use and close the bathroom door before flushing the toilet.

Feng shui experts believe that bathrooms arranged en suite with a bedroom are undesirable because the flushing or draining of water disturbs the chi in the bedroom.

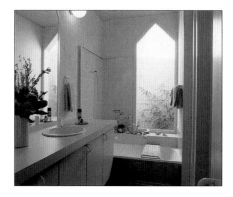

PREVENTING STAGNATION
Hard, smooth, and reflective materials speed up the flow of chi, which reduces the risk of its stagnating. This bathroom has mirrors, tiles, plants, and natural light to stimulate chi.

S

SE   SW

IDEAL POSITION

E   East or southeast   W
to take full
advantage of
available morning
sunlight to keep
the room dry.

NE   NW

N

BEDROOM

Because we spend so much time in a bedroom sleeping, feng shui practitioners believe that carefully locating and arranging bedrooms can help us align ourselves with the flow of energy in a way that enhances our waking life.

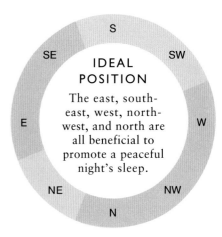

IDEAL POSITION

The east, southeast, west, northwest, and north are all beneficial to promote a peaceful night's sleep.

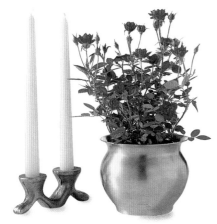

ENCOURAGING ROMANCE
Decor can do much to encourage romance. Red is the color of passion, so red flowers are beneficial; paired objects, such as two plants in a pot, reinforce relationships, while candles encourage the fire energy associated with passion.

Bed Directions

The position of your bed in a room makes a difference to energy flow. Your head pointing northwest can help you feel more in control and gain a sense of leadership. For young people the head pointing east can help to build careers and stimulate growth. The west can both encourage good sleep and be beneficial for romance. Bad directions in which to place the head of your bed include northeast, which can make you feel edgy and may cause nightmares, and south, which is too hot and fiery and can lead to arguments.

The bedroom often fulfills several functions, but above all it should be a calm place where you can have a peaceful night's sleep. If you are an insomniac or have trouble sleeping, it is recommended that you locate the bedroom on the north side of the house because this direction is characterized by more peaceful, quieter chi. However, it is also important to feel energized in the morning; if you lack sufficient energy at the start of the day, a bedroom facing east can offset this problem.

The bedroom is also a place of intimacy, and fostering a sense of romance, along with privacy, is important. If you feel that your love life is in need of a boost, feng shui suggests locating the bedroom to the west, which is a favorable position for encouraging pleasure and romance. A bedroom positioned in the northwest can be ideal for parents because the chi here can encourage better control of one's life and help to develop wisdom.

Wall-to-wall carpet and softly draped curtains are suggested for bedrooms because they slow chi and create a relaxing atmosphere. Bed linens of natural fibers, such as cotton, create a good energy flow against the skin, and it is recommended that you always make the bed in the morning.

BEDROOM COLORS
Feng shui practitioners believe that a background of white, cream, or pale tones of pink or gray encourage the flow of chi.

A wood-framed bed has a neutral effect on chi. In feng shui terms, futons are ideal beds because they have a wooden frame and the mattress is made of natural materials—four to eight layers of cotton wadding bound by a strong cotton cover—which help to promote sound and restful sleep.

Followers of feng shui advise that you should be able to see the door and window of your bedroom from your bed.

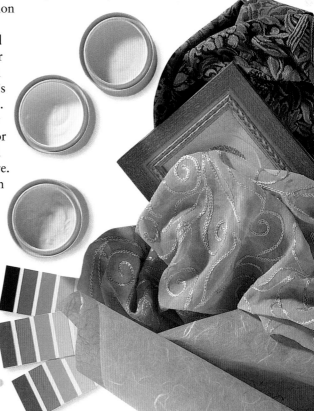

A CHILD'S ROOM

Children's bedrooms are usually a place both of rest and play. The aim should be to help them sleep soundly at night while stimulating and encouraging their growth and development during the day.

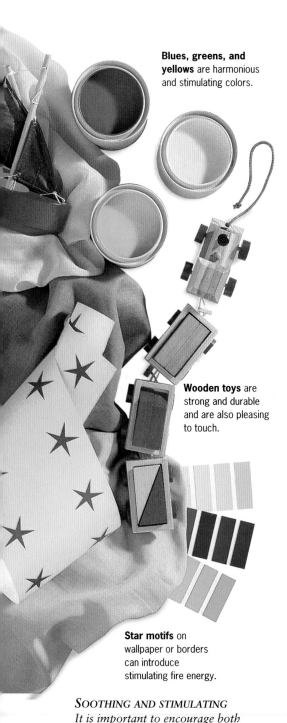

Blues, greens, and yellows are harmonious and stimulating colors.

Wooden toys are strong and durable and are also pleasing to touch.

Star motifs on wallpaper or borders can introduce stimulating fire energy.

SOOTHING AND STIMULATING
It is important to encourage both stimulation and a sense of calm in a child's room. Plain walls and furnishings in bright colors are stimulating, and the gentle movement of a mobile can be useful in promoting a peaceful atmosphere.

The ideal position for a child's room is in the east or southeast. The east is associated with youthful energy, and it encourages growth; however, it may be too stimulating for sleep. The southeast may be preferable because while it also promotes activity, the energy is gentler.

If two children are sharing a room, there may be occasional friction and arguments. It is important for each child to have some personal space, so try to provide each youngster with at least one personal shelf or drawer. Bed positions can also encourage harmony; feng shui recommends placing the beds of both children in the same direction. If your relations with one child are strained, try situating your own bed in the same direction as his or hers.

Problems in sleeping can occur in both babies and children. If you can, place the bassinet or crib so that the child's head is facing north. There are certain directions in which you should definitely not place your child's bed. The northeast could cause tantrums; the south may be disturbing; and the southwest could lead to timidity. If you have a child who is particularly anxious or hyperactive, consider putting this child in a bedroom that faces west. It is characterized by calm, contented energy, which can help settle a child.

Using yang colors, such as red, pink, or bright yellow, can add a touch of energy. Natural wood is a good option for the floor of any child's room because it provides stimulating chi and is also easily cleaned. Fabric blinds are a good choice for window coverings because they can be completely closed at night, slowing chi, but can be fully rolled up during the day to let in maximum natural light. Make sure there is plenty of storage space for toys and books to avoid clutter.

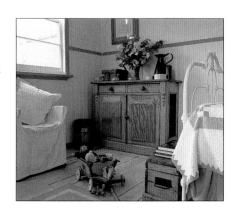

DECOR FOR A CHILD'S ROOM
This bedroom follows many feng shui principles. The wood floor, the decor of blue and yellow, and the wooden toys and toy box encourage a healthy flow of chi to stimulate the child.

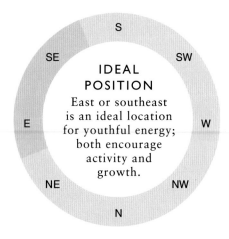

IDEAL POSITION
East or southeast is an ideal location for youthful energy; both encourage activity and growth.

S
SE
SW
E
W
NE
NW
N

CHAPTER 5

THE WORKING ENVIRONMENT

*Most of us spend at least one-third of our
day at work, so we need to be conscious of the
health of the environment there. Many workplaces,
whether in the industrial, office, or service sector,
harbor potential hazards, some of which are easier to
identify and deal with than others. But we all need
to take responsibility for spotting dangers in the
working environment and do our part to control
them before they can cause a serious problem.*

THE IMPORTANCE OF A HEALTHY WORKPLACE

Wherever you work and whatever time you spend there, it is worth doing all you can to ensure that your working environment is a healthy and safe one.

Good working conditions are a boon to the health of employees and their employers as well. In an unhealthy working environment people are more likely to suffer ill health and be less productive. Poor working conditions can seriously undermine the success of a business because of absenteeism due to illness.

Large-scale disasters on the job are fortunately rare, but when they do occur, they can be very costly in terms of lives and money. One example is the Piper Alpha explosion in the North Sea in 1988, which cost 167 lives and an estimated $1.3 billion.

In 1997 in the United States, as many as 6,200 people lost their lives in on-the-job accidents, another 60,000 died from work-related illnesses and injuries, and some 6 million suffered occupational illnesses and injuries. Worldwide, loss of life through work-related illnesses and injuries amounted to 2 million people that year.

A HEALTHY WORKPLACE

Good occupational health management is about ensuring that a job does not jeopardize the health of any workers and that employees are fit for the task. Health risks

---

THE MODERN WORKING ENVIRONMENT

Over the past 20 years there has been a revolution in the way both employers and employees regard their workplace. Many forward-thinking companies have recognized the importance of providing a pleasant, safe, and harmonious workplace, which can reduce staff turnover and improve productivity.

Feng shui principles have been applied in a number of new office developments. More companies are recognizing that open space, bright light, and greenery help to create a sense of harmony.

Fitness centers have been incorporated into many new office complexes so that employees can take advantage of free time at lunch or after work to get fit and reduce stress.

Annual health checks are provided by many large corporations, and moderate-size and large companies also offer health insurance at reduced rates.

Staff restaurants have been revolutionized in many workplaces. They now offer a variety of choices to suit many tastes and include healthful options.

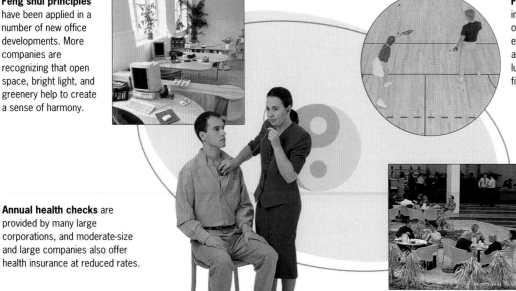

UNCOVERING HEALTH HAZARDS ON THE JOB

Before taking a new job, it makes sense to ask some basic questions that pertain to health and safety issues in your new workplace. If you are aware of potential health problems, you may be able to take some preventive actions.

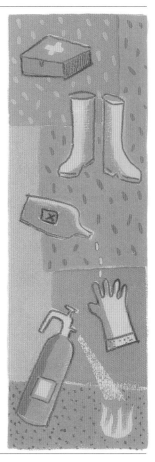

QUESTIONS TO ASK A POTENTIAL EMPLOYER

1. Will I come into contact with harmful or excessive dusts, fumes, gases, or vapors?

2. Will I work with radioactive materials, microwaves, or lasers?

3. Will I be exposed to drugs, hormones, molds, parasites, bacteria, animals, or animal products?

4. Are some materials likely to cause skin irritation? If so, will I need to take protective measures?

5. Is all machinery in good working order?

6. What sort of training and safety instruction do employees receive?

7. Will I be exposed to excessive noise?

8. Are there ventilation systems to extract dangerous dusts and fumes?

9. Are there adequate monitoring systems to detect dangerous leakage of chemicals?

10. Should I wear any form of protective clothing?

11. Are fire precautions in place?

12. Is first-aid equipment available?

in the workplace come in many forms. Handling heavy goods can cause musculoskeletal injuries, such as a back spasm; inhaling hazardous substances can lead to asthma and respiratory diseases, such as asbestosis; exposure to high noise levels can impair hearing; and excessive vibrations can cause nerve and bone damage.

Employers are duty bound under health and safety legislation to identify and control health risks that arise at work and must establish safety procedures for all their employees. But unless there are adequate monitoring procedures and fines for violations, many hazards may not be dealt with adequately. Employees and unions must also be willing to confront companies that have violations and be willing to work with them to correct problems.

The nature of hazards in many modern workplaces has changed; employees today are more often concerned about poor ventilation or high levels of stress in the workplace than physical injury. Although we know that prolonged stress can lead to high blood pressure, heart disease, and depression, linking such conditions purely to work

stress is difficult. Nevertheless, most enlightened employers realize that it pays to invest in the health of their employees. Making certain that lighting is adequate, the temperature is comfortable, and indoor air pollutants and distracting noise are kept to a minimum contributes to employee health. Simple provisions, such as fitness activities and weight reduction programs on site and annual health checks for staff, can also make the workforce fitter and more motivated.

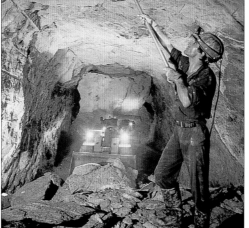

HIGH-RISK WORK
Quarrying and mining are particularly hazardous occupations. Workers are exposed to all sorts of risks, including toxic dust, excessive noise, and physical injury. Adequate protection, such as headgear, is essential, and employees should carefully follow all safety instructions.

115

HAZARDS IN THE WORKPLACE

Any workplace may contain hazards. Understanding the dangers in your own working environment will help you to minimize possible risks; care and attention are the keystones.

Every adult who is employed full-time spends more than half of his or her waking hours in the workplace. Having a safe and healthy environment there is as important as it is at home. Many of the job dangers routinely endured by previous generations, especially in the industrial factories and sweat shops of the 19th century, have largely been eliminated in the Western world, but other concerns, such as stress and contamination from toxic chemicals, have arisen. Even if an employer takes care to ensure that the working environment is safe, it is important for all employees to be aware of potential dangers and to conduct themselves safely at work.

OFFICES

An office may seem to offer the ultimate safe working environment. But while the magnitude of risk is obviously not as high as that in a foundry, mine, or construction

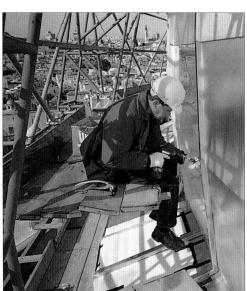

site, office premises can nevertheless present significant hazards to employees (see page 119). Slipping, tripping, and falling are the greatest causes of serious injury in the office. Yet taking precautions against such accidents is usually fairly simple and, by and large, a matter of common sense. Any spills should be cleaned up immediately, and corridors should be kept clear of boxes, tables, files, and other paraphernalia. All staircases should have securely fixed handrails. You should avoid carrying large and awkward loads around the office; it is better to make several trips, use a dolly, or ask for some help to move equipment or bulky objects.

Filing cabinet drawers should never be left open unattended; they could injure a person who is not looking where he or she is walking. Also, you should never open more than one drawer of a filing cabinet at a time because the cabinet will become unstable and it might topple over on someone. (Most filing cabinets are designed to prevent this occurrence, but some old models still in use may not have this feature.) Since filing cabinets are very heavy, such an accident could cause severe injury. Also, electrical cables and extension cords should never be trailed across the floor where they can easily be tripped over.

In many offices, space is at a premium, and any available floor space is soon filled. In addition to making the office environment claustrophobic, this situation can lead to unsafe, unsecured stacking and storage of equipment. Very often the only way to store items is to stack them upward, and as a result, some materials and files may be accessible only by ladder or footstool. Taking a shortcut, such as standing on a chair to reach items, could lead to a fall. To avoid

FENG SHUI FOR YOUR DESKTOP

You can apply feng shui principles to your desk, arranging items to maximize positive energy, but you must first determine in which direction your desk faces. Establish magnetic north, then find the center of the desk and place a grid of the eight directions over it (see page 105). Each direction is associated with a particular form of energy that can have positive benefits on your work.

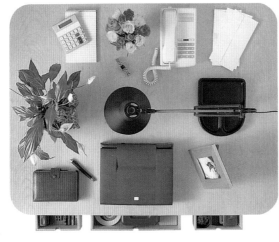

Northeast encourages motivation; place objects here that encourage you to work harder, such as your appointment calendar.

North encourages tranquillity; if your workplace is hectic, placing a plant or flowers here can promote calmness.

Southeast encourages communication; the telephone, the fax if you have one, and your mail tray would be well placed here.

Southwest encourages family harmony; this spot is ideal for family photographs or mementos.

DESKTOP ENERGY
Your desk must be large enough for your needs. Rounded corners and pale wood encourage the flow of chi.

West is associated with finance, so checkbooks and petty cash boxes sit well in this location.

this possibility, make sure that all items used on a daily basis are easily accessed and that there is proper equipment for reaching out-of-the-way items.

Office work can give rise to a number of problems and complaints, such as stress, muscular problems from poor seating posture or repetitive strain, hearing difficulties, eye problems, and increased incidences of colds and flu. Proper ventilation, effective lighting, and ergonomic arrangements that allow workers to interact safely and efficiently with their environment help to create a comfortable and productive workplace.

Electronic equipment at work

The personal computer not only has revolutionized the way we work in offices but has also led to a shift in the nature of health problems encountered by office workers, most notably eyestrain and carpal tunnel syndrome—a condition of the hand and wrist characterized by persistent numbness, burning, and tingling due to repeating the same motions over and over. Preventive action is the best way to avoid such problems (see pages 61 and 124–126).

One piece of equipment that can cause health risks if not used properly is the photocopier (see page 118). There has been a great deal of speculation about the potential hazards arising from radiation emitted by photocopiers, but in fact the biggest hazard associated with them is electricity. Untrained employees should never attempt to adjust or repair a machine, and everyone should understand and follow usage instructions.

The inside of a photocopier can be very hot; if it has to be opened—for example, to clear a paper jam—this should be done very carefully. Also, employees should wash their hands thoroughly if they come into contact with the toner, which is toxic.

Two other hazards associated with photocopiers are the photocopying light bar and the generation of ozone gas. Neither of these is a significant risk, however, if sensible precautions are taken. Photocopying should be done with the lid down whenever possible, and the person using the machine should look away from the light to prevent damage to the eyes. Also, the machine should be located in a well-ventilated and reasonably sized room to prevent the buildup of ozone, which is potentially lethal.

FENG SHUI STORAGE
Offices generate clutter, which can obstruct clear thinking and productivity. One way to maintain control is to use mini storage units to keep paraphernalia, such as pens and paper clips, neatly tucked away.

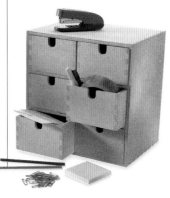

FACTORIES

Industrial premises take many different forms and can present different types of hazards. Although in most Western countries the size of the heavy industrial sector is diminishing and softer, cleaner technologies are emerging, it is clear that factories still pose the threat of major accidents or ill health. Heavy machinery, large volumes of dangerous substances, and the use of huge amounts of energy—thermal, electrical, and/or chemical—create a potentially hazardous situation.

The majority of modern machines are constructed or supplied with protection devices to prevent operators from becoming trapped or caught up in moving parts. For example, electrosensitive sensors will warn employees if they are dangerously close to moving parts. A large proportion of accidents occur when machinery is being cleaned or maintained. There are several reasons for this. Guards often have to be removed so that normally inaccessible parts can be worked on; in this circumstance the power to the machinery should be isolated or completely cut off if possible. Also, maintenance personnel are often employed on a contract basis and may not be familiar with the working conditions of a particular factory. And cleaning may involve the use of hazardous substances that, if used in confined spaces, could cause health problems. If you have to clean or maintain equipment, be extra vigilant about safety.

Chemicals and other substances

Many industries use a number of hazardous substances that are capable of causing a variety of health problems. Some problems may emerge quickly, but others can build up over time. For example, inhaling a very high concentration of certain chemicals can be fatal after only a few breaths, whereas inhaling asbestos may cause lung disease many years later. Exposure to chromate compounds can cause skin ulcers in the short term and may lead to skin cancer after a longer period. Substances that are hazardous to health are labeled variously as very toxic, toxic, harmful, or irritant.

There are other potentially hazardous substances encountered in the workplace besides chemicals. These include dust, microorganisms, and fumes, which may be given off by raw materials, an intermediate

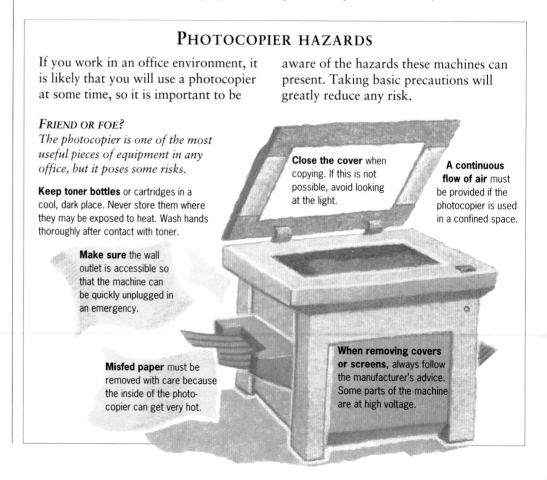

PHOTOCOPIER HAZARDS

If you work in an office environment, it is likely that you will use a photocopier at some time, so it is important to be aware of the hazards these machines can present. Taking basic precautions will greatly reduce any risk.

FRIEND OR FOE?
The photocopier is one of the most useful pieces of equipment in any office, but it poses some risks.

Keep toner bottles or cartridges in a cool, dark place. Never store them where they may be exposed to heat. Wash hands thoroughly after contact with toner.

Make sure the wall outlet is accessible so that the machine can be quickly unplugged in an emergency.

Misfed paper must be removed with care because the inside of the photocopier can get very hot.

Close the cover when copying. If this is not possible, avoid looking at the light.

A continuous flow of air must be provided if the photocopier is used in a confined space.

When removing covers or screens, always follow the manufacturer's advice. Some parts of the machine are at high voltage.

CHEMICAL HAZARDS IN AN OFFICE ENVIRONMENT

Certain chemicals common to many workplaces are potentially harmful. The table below lists some of these chemicals, the products in which they are found, their possible effects, and what you should do if you are exposed to them.

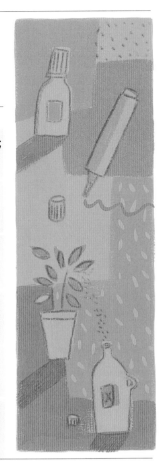

SOURCE	CHEMICAL NAME	EFFECTS	COPING STRATEGIES
Photocopiers	Ozone, solvents in the toner	Coughs, chest pain, shortness of breath, eye irritation, and nausea	Provide good ventilation; wash hands thoroughly after contact with toner.
Correction fluids	Trichloroethane, trichloroethylene	Fatigue, depression, and memory loss if inhaled in large doses	Increase ventilation; use correction tapes whenever possible.
Glue	Phenol, ethanol, formaldehyde, propanol, acetone	Eye irritation and breathing difficulties	Increase ventilation; use sticky tapes and nontoxic glues.
Furniture, shelves, carpeting, upholstery	Formaldehyde in particle-board and furnishings	Eye irritation, headache, and drowsiness	Seal furniture and shelves with nontoxic varnish.
Marker pens	Acetone, ammonia, benzyl alcohol, toluene, xylene	Drowsiness, headache, confusion, and nausea if inhaled in large doses	Use water-based pens; increase ventilation.
Office cleaning products	Phenol, dinitrobenzene	Skin irritation and headaches	Use nontoxic, natural products for cleaning furniture and machines.

product, the final products, or the by-products and waste from the manufacturing process. Assessments of any risks should be carried out during each stage of production.

Hazardous substances come in several forms—solid, liquid, gas, and vapor (given off by solids or liquids). People can be badly affected by the inhalation of dust, gases, or vapors; for example, exposure to cadmium dust or fumes can cause lung disease and even kidney damage. Workers can also be affected by the ingestion of solids, dust, and liquids; for example, exposure to inorganic mercury salts can cause mercury poisoning. An employee whose skin has come into contact with some harmful or irritant substances can develop burns or contact dermatitis or, in extreme cases, more complicated internal problems.

The risks to health posed by dangerous substances depend on their potency and the level and length of exposure to them. Exposure limits for most known hazardous substances have been established. It is up to the employer to make sure they are not exceeded in the workplace and that all risks are properly managed throughout the produc-

tion process. Employees must do their part as well by carefully following all health and safety instructions issued to them.

CONSTRUCTION SITES

The nature and conditions of the construction industry make it one of the most hazardous fields of occupation. Much about the business is inherently dangerous, and extensive planning and organization are required when a construction project is being set up to make sure that the health, safety, and welfare of all employees are built into the process from the outset. Excavating and working at a great height are often requirements of construction work. All aspects of the process present risks to construction workers in different ways.

Falls are the largest cause of accidental death in the construction industry. Yet most accidents involving falls can be avoided if the right equipment is provided and properly used. If it is possible to fall more than six feet from the edge of any working platform, access route, or stairway, there must be guard rails or other suitable barriers for protection.

CONSTRUCTION DANGERS: LESSONS FOR US ALL

Construction work is one of the most dangerous occupations, but many of the specific problems faced could apply to anyone, both at home and at work.

▶ *Injuries, especially of the back, are common, the result of falling or incorrectly lifting a heavy object. When moving cumbersome objects, it is best to use a dolly or wheeled trolley. If you must lift a heavy item manually, bend from the knees so that the leg muscles do the work instead of the back.*

▶ *Construction workers must often sit or stand in awkward positions for long periods and are therefore prone to muscle and tendon strain. Taking breaks and changing positions frequently will help prevent injury.*

▶ *Mishaps with ladders are common. Avoid working alone on a ladder; always have another person nearby to brace a ladder for you and to hand you tools and materials.*

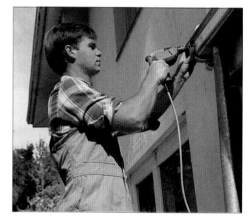

SAFETY ON THE JOB
Construction jobs often involve the use of a hand drill for extended periods. This repetitive and often strenuous action can place excess strain on muscles and joints. It is important to take regular breaks.

LADDER SAFETY
Always follow basic safety procedures on a ladder and make sure that it is in good repair and well secured. Step-ladders must be fully extended, with supporting crossbars locked in place.

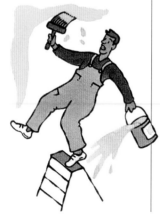

Ladders are generally suitable only for light work and then only if the work can be done without overstretching. They must be braced to prevent their slipping and must have a good handhold for the worker. No matter what precautions are taken, working on ladders is still dangerous; a large proportion of ladder accidents happen during work that lasts less than 30 minutes. The longer the ladder, the more problems there are in using it safely. Ladders longer than 30 feet should be used as a means of access only in extreme circumstances.

Scaffolding, which is used as a working platform, should be based on a firm and level foundation and be stabilized with sturdy supports or by bracing it to a building. Scaffolding should be capable of supporting the load it is designed to hold, taking into account any weathering stresses, and the boards should be arranged to avoid tipping and tripping. Regular inspection should be carried out to ensure that it remains safe.

If necessary, safety harnesses can be worn by workers to provide extra protection at great heights. A harness will not prevent a fall but will minimize the risk of injury if someone does fall. When a harness is used, the possible fall with it should not be greater than six feet, and consideration must also be given to how an employee who falls can be easily and safely recovered.

Work below ground on a building site can also be hazardous. Sometimes injuries are caused by accidental contact with underground service conduits, such as electrical cables or gas pipelines. Therefore, it is absolutely essential that excavation work be properly planned and carefully carried out; the sides of a site must be kept stable, and there should be no danger of materials falling onto people working below ground. Accounting for the vibrations from blasting and the movement of heavy equipment around the site is also important because vibrations from vehicles or dynamite could cause a collapse of unstable earth or weaken the foundations of nearby structures.

The following is a checklist that construction managers are asked to consider in order to ensure the safety of workers.

▶ Working areas and walkways are level and free from obstructions.

▶ Holes are securely fenced or covered.

▶ Materials are stored safely.

▶ Nails in lumber from demolition are removed or hammered down.

▶ Adequate lighting is provided for work in the dark or a poor light situation.

▶ Props or shores are put in place to make structures safe.

▶ All waste is collected and disposed of properly.

OTHER WORKPLACE PROBLEMS

Although a number of problems in the workplace are specific to certain jobs, some aspects of a working environment can cause difficulties in a whole spectrum of professions.

Every occupation carries some element of risk to health. While many of these problems are easily prevented—by wearing appropriate protective gear when handling toxic chemicals, for example, or by not lifting loads that are too heavy—others can be more difficult to combat.

SICK BUILDING SYNDROME

Almost everyone occasionally feels unwell, suffering from one or more common symptoms of discomfort, such as headache, dry throat, or sore eyes. Sick building syndrome describes a situation in which, for no easily

identifiable reason, people working in a particular building experience such symptoms on a regular basis. If illness is caused by the building, symptoms tend to increase in severity the longer a person spends time at work, and the symptoms improve or disappear once the sufferer has been away from the building for a few days.

The main symptoms associated with sick building syndrome are dry or itchy eyes, nose, or throat; a stuffy or runny nose; dry, itchy skin or a rash; headache; lethargy; irritability; and poor ability to concentrate. The symptoms are often mild and do not

MEASURING CHRONIC STRESS

Employers have increasingly been forced to recognize that workplace conditions can cause chronic stress, which is harmful in the long run. Until recently, however, there has been no reliable method for measuring stress levels. One method that was often used tracked hormonal imbalances, but because stress hormones tend to fluctuate throughout the day, the tests could be unreliable. The newer Adrenal Stress Index test measures hormonal imbalances in samples of saliva. The samples can be taken throughout a

normal day, which is essential for measuring the daily fluctuations of the two hormones most indicative of the long-term effects of stress: cortisol and dehydro-epiandosterone (DHEA).

HORMONAL FLUCTUATION
After rising in response to stress, a healthy person's hormone levels quickly return to normal. In a chronically stressed person, however, the level of cortisol remains high, even after the cause of the stress has been removed.

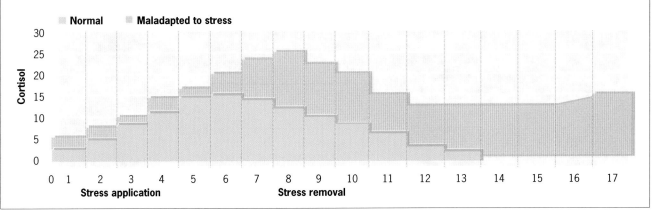

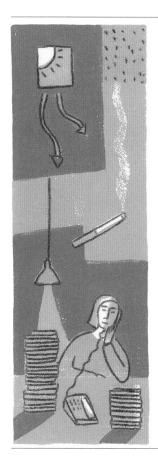

COPING WITH SICK BUILDING SYNDROME

It is especially difficult to find the cause of and to remedy sick building syndrome, but there are certain steps you can take to improve your immediate working area if you suspect that your building is making you sick. Also, management can log all complaints in a building performance database to help locate problems.

SYMPTOMS

Dry, itchy eyes, nose, and throat; stuffy or runny nose; dry, itchy skin or rash; headache; lethargy; irritability; poor ability to concentrate.

REMEDIES

Try to improve ventilation in your area. If you are able to open a nearby window, do so on a regular basis. Even if you open windows only at the beginning and end of the day, you will help rid your area of stale air and reduce the impact of irritants that can cause dry, itchy eyes and a stuffy nose.

If you are a manager, make sure that the heating and air-conditioning system is properly maintained, the ducts are cleaned regularly, and none of the air vents is blocked. Have an air quality survey done every year or two.

Bring plants into your work area. A few, like golden pothos and spider plant, are known to absorb pollutants that may cause headaches, lethargy, and other symptoms. Other kinds of plants at least add life and modulate dry air.

Try to improve your outlook and sense of control in the workplace. Maintain a positive attitude and work toward solving any job-related problems by discussing your role in the workplace with your managers. Use stress-reduction techniques, such as meditation, because stress can aggravate any adverse physical condition.

If your work area is insufficiently cleaned, notify the managers so they can see to it that the cleaning service is doing its job efficiently. Organize office cleanup days to get rid of unneeded materials that are collecting dust.

appear to cause any lasting damage. However, to people suffering from them, such symptoms are far from trivial and can cause considerable distress. In severe cases they can affect a person's ability to work and may represent a significant cost to business in the form of reduced staff efficiency, increased absenteeism and staff turnover, extended work breaks, and reduced overtime, as well as time lost while supervisors try to deal with complaints.

Cases of sick building syndrome started to appear in the 1970s, when concerns about fuel shortages inspired architects and building contractors to design or remodel buildings with good insulation and sealed windows to conserve energy. By 1982 the World Health Organization was estimating that as many as 30 percent of new and remodeled buildings were involved in the phenomenon worldwide.

Sick building syndrome is not a recognized illness but a convenient term to describe something that cannot be diagnosed precisely. It should not be confused with specific illnesses associated with problems in an air-conditioning system, such as Legionnaires' disease, or exposure to toxic substances, such as formaldehyde. Nor does it cover the effects of adverse physical conditions in the workplace—excessive noise or extremes of heat or cold, for instance.

Despite extensive research, the exact causes of sick building syndrome are still not known, but it appears that a combination of factors is responsible, and the relative importance of factors within a combination may be different in each case. Broadly, these factors fall into two categories—physical and emotional. Physical, or environmental, conditions include ventilation, cleaning and maintenance practices, and the layout of workstations. The emotional aspects may be related to employees' feelings about their jobs, including a lack of variety or absorbing interest or the inability to control certain aspects of the job and working environment.

The conditions believed to cause sick building syndrome are usually interrelated. For example, poorly maintained air-conditioning systems can create problems not only with ventilation but also with temperature and humidity control; new furnishings that release chemical pollutants into the air and insufficient or badly organized cleaning services can create or intensify problems related to dust and toxic fumes. Environmental problems can be exacerbated further by low job satisfaction. Not all the possible factors occur in every case, nor do symptoms necessarily appear if any of the conditions are present. It is likely that factors combine in certain ways to create the kind of environmental and working stress in which sick building syndrome occurs.

Almost any building can be affected by sick building syndrome. There have been reports of outbreaks in many different types of structures, including hospitals and even some homes. In general, however, the problem seems to be most common in large office buildings that have automated ventilation systems and sealed windows.

Workers most commonly affected by the symptoms tend to be those who have little control over their working environment and who are employed in routine jobs, such as general clerical work or computer data entry. Women seem to be more at risk than men, but this can be partly explained by the fact that more women are employed in the highest risk areas.

Many of the factors associated with sick building syndrome seem to relate to the design and the materials used in construction. In most cases it would be difficult, if not impossible, to change physical aspects of the building once construction and installation work have been completed. In some instances alteration might be possible but would be far too expensive to be feasible. The prevention of sick building syndrome, therefore, needs to be tackled at an early stage during the planning of a new building or the remodeling or change of use of an older one. For example, the intake for fresh air should not be located in a garage or near a traffic light where cars will be idling.

NOISE AT WORK

Despite rapid technological progress and changing employment patterns, hundreds of thousands of workers are exposed every day to loud noise at work, which may be damaging to their health. In Britain alone, it is estimated that between 500,000 and 1 million workers are exposed every day to noise levels of about 90 decibels (db) for periods of up to 8 hours, while as many as 2 million workers may be exposed to noise levels of about 84 db. All workers exposed to noise levels in this range run some risk of suffering from permanent noise-induced hearing loss. While employees in especially noisy trades continue to develop serious occupational deafness, many more people at work suffer from hearing loss in less acute forms, which is nonetheless distressing, both physically and socially.

People working in conditions noisy enough to induce temporary hearing loss—that is, continuous noise above 80 db—can expect a permanent loss to the same degree after being exposed to these conditions for about 10 years. Recovery from temporary hearing loss usually takes a few hours or at most a couple of days if the noise exposure has been severe.

Continuous loud noise rarely hurts the eardrum or the little bones in the middle ear, but the sensitive hair cells in the inner ear can be affected. These cells are killed by continuous loud noise. The damage is irreversible, and the cells cannot be replaced.

Noise not only damages hearing sensitivity but can also give rise to tinnitus—a disturbing sound, such as ringing, buzzing, whistling, humming, or roaring, in the ears. This condition is especially troublesome at night, when it can prevent sleep. Recent research explains tinnitus as the exaggerated reverberation of the hair cells' response to sound; it is actually an echo of our own hearing mechanism.

Besides causing temporary or permanent hearing loss, noise can also be a safety hazard. Most obviously, noise interferes with verbal communication, leading to errors and failures to respond to warning sounds or shouts. This is, of course, made worse in situations where individuals have grown accustomed to noise as a result of temporary or permanent hearing loss. Such deafness can not only affect workplace safety

SOUNDPROOFING YOUR WORK AREA

Open-plan offices are increasingly common, but they can present noise problems. At best you may be continually distracted by interruptions; at worst you may suffer from stress. There are a number of steps you can take to reduce the impact of noise.

▶ *Sound bounces around in empty spaces. Create some sound absorption features with plants, bulletin boards, bookcases, or files.*

▶ *Create a visual barrier. Often the impact of noise is reduced by visual barriers, helping to suggest an enclosed and private space.*

▶ *Be assertive about your need for quiet. At times everyone needs some silence. If you make your colleagues aware of your needs they will probably cooperate with you.*

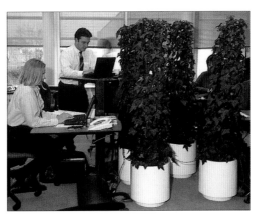

PLANT POWER
Office plants are effective at absorbing noise and pollutants and providing privacy. They also add color and life to an office environment.

REPETITIVE STRESS INJURY

Repetitive stress injury covers several complaints caused by a repetitive action. People who work at computer keyboards for long periods are particularly vulnerable. The tendons in the forearm become inflamed, resulting in tenosynovitis or carpal tunnel syndrome and severe pain. Wrist splints may help temporarily, but most workplaces now recognize that well-designed workstations and regular breaks are essential preventive measures.

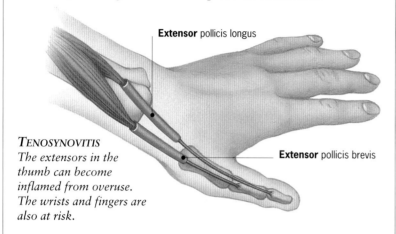

Extensor pollicis longus

TENOSYNOVITIS
The extensors in the thumb can become inflamed from overuse. The wrists and fingers are also at risk.

Extensor pollicis brevis

but may also affect the safety of an individual outside the workplace. Increased noise levels and stress are clearly related. High levels of noise can be distracting and lower workers' levels of concentration. This in turn can lead to an increase in stress and to errors, which in some circumstances can have safety implications of their own.

UPPER LIMB DISORDERS

Many disorders of the upper limbs can be caused or made worse by work activities. Various parts of the limbs may be affected, but it is usually the tendons, which connect muscles to bones, the muscles themselves, and the associated nerve supply that cause concern. Severity may range from occasional aches and other discomfort of the affected part to well-defined cases of disease or injury. Loss of function can also occur, resulting in a reduced ability to work.

Links between certain work activities and upper limb disorders have long been recognized. Early examples include cotton twister's wrist and telegrapher's cramp. Although automation has reduced the prevalence of these conditions, upper limb disorders still account for a considerable amount of occupational ill health and are not specific to one particular sector.

Although many symptoms are associated with upper limb disorders, the most notable are pain, restriction of joint movement, and swelling. In some conditions the sense of touch is diminished and manual dexterity is reduced. If the onset of symptoms is gradual, the body may overcompensate for the problem, causing further damage to the limb and possibly even permanent disability.

Forceful repetitive movements over an extended period are associated with the onset of upper limb disorders; examples of such movements include gripping, twisting, or reaching with the hand. And if the movements are awkward to perform, they can worsen the problem. At present researchers are unable to set precise limits for any of the various factors because their interaction is not sufficiently understood. However, you should consider these risks and take regular breaks from repetitive work activities.

Carpal tunnel syndrome

Carpal tunnel syndrome, a type of repetitive stress injury, affects the hands and wrists and is the most common hand problem that primary care physicians see. It has been estimated that millions of Americans have the syndrome, mostly as a result of their work.

The typical symptoms are persistent numbness, burning, and tingling of the hands, as if they had fallen asleep. Many people also experience stiffness and swelling in their wrists and loss of hand strength and dexterity, especially when doing a task that requires fine movement, such as sewing.

The cause is inflammation or swelling of the median nerve, which carries messages between the hand and brain. This nerve passes through the carpal tunnel, a narrow opening on the palm side of the wrist through which nine tendons also pass. If one or more of these tendons swells or an injury causes the space inside the tunnel to narrow, the nerve may become pinched or irritated, leading to the characteristic symptoms.

Computer operators, pianists, meat packers, and jackhammer operators are among those who have a high risk of carpal tunnel syndrome. Treatment usually involves rest and immobilization of the affected hand and wrist and sometimes a splint to hold the wrist in a straight, unflexed position. Alternative therapies can also be helpful. An acupuncturist may stimulate the meridians affecting the neck, back, and shoulders, as well as those of the hands, wrists, and arms, in order to heal the entire length of the injured nerve. A chiropractor may adjust not only the wrist but also the areas where the median nerve is connected with the rest of the nervous system, including the arm, shoulder, and neck. Many chiropractors and some acupuncturists also use transcutaneous nerve stimulation, or TENS, the application of mild electrical pulses to the skin that causes the body to produce endorphins—its natural painkillers. A practitioner of Alexander technique can also help by assessing posture and habitual movements and suggesting changes to correct habits that are contributing to the syndrome.

WORKPLACE LIGHTING

Good lighting, whether natural or artificial, is a very important part of health and safety at work. It helps people to see and avoid hazards and reduces occurrences of visual fatigue and discomfort—an important consideration in many forms of work.

In all working and access areas, workers must be able to see well enough to avoid tripping, falling, or walking into obstacles. In addition, some jobs require the ability to see fine detail. For example, operators of machinery may need to see a workpiece from a distance or to read gauges and displays accurately. The level and type of lighting needed for safety in working areas therefore depend on the type of work being done and the hazards associated with it.

Several difficulties can arise from inadequate or inappropriate lighting. Glare, for instance, can cause problems at two different levels. At the disability level, glare directly interferes with vision and affects the sensitivity of the visual system. Driving at night toward a car with its headlights on full beam is a common example; glare can make objects next to or beyond the car very difficult to see. At the discomfort level, glare can cause general unease, annoyance, irritability, or distraction from your work, but it does not directly impair your vision. On the other hand, overly intense light can cause tissue damage.

Although healthy eyes cannot actually be strained by overuse, poor lighting can lead to visual fatigue, or what we call eyestrain, because eyes have to work harder in order to see properly. The symptoms of eyestrain vary according to lighting conditions and the task being carried out. They are likely to occur whenever your eyes have to act at the limits of their capabilities for an extended period of time. Eyestrain is not caused only by poor lighting. It is inevitable if you are farsighted or nearsighted and do not wear glasses to correct your vision. Symptoms include irritation and inflammation of the eyes and eyelids, itchiness, blurred or double vision, headaches, fatigue, and dizziness.

Poor lighting can also have other, more indirect effects on general health. The natural response to insufficient light is to get closer to the task at hand or to look at it from a different, perhaps awkward direction. This can lead to adopting unusual or strained postures that can cause backache and other signs of strain.

There have been a few reports that exposure to fluorescent lights may be linked to the development of malignant melanoma, a relatively uncommon but serious form of skin cancer. However, current evidence does not support this claim. Fluorescent lights are low-pressure mercury discharge lamps that generate ultraviolet radiation internally. Most of the ultraviolet radiation is absorbed

Creative recycling

Decoupage, which literally means "cutting out," refers to the practice of decorating things with printed paper or cards. It is a simple, creative way of recycling old greeting cards or magazines, which you can use for decorating items in your office to personalize them and give them a fresh, original look.

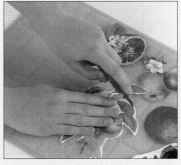

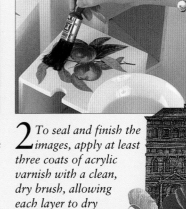

1 *Choose your decorative images and carefully cut out the motifs with a craft knife. Glue these onto the object to be decorated and press down firmly. Use a damp sponge to wipe off any excess glue, and allow to dry.*

2 *To seal and finish the images, apply at least three coats of acrylic varnish with a clean, dry brush, allowing each layer to dry thoroughly.*

USE YOUR COMPUTER SAFELY

A number of accessories are available that are specifically designed to protect your health from the various hazards of computers. Ergonomic keyboards may look outlandish when compared with traditional keyboards, but in fact they have been designed to better suit the natural actions of the hands. Wrist support pads help to keep your wrists in alignment with your hands as you type, easing the muscular and tendon strain that can cause carpal tunnel syndrome. And screen guards, which reduce the glare from monitors can help to ease eyestrain and prevent headaches.

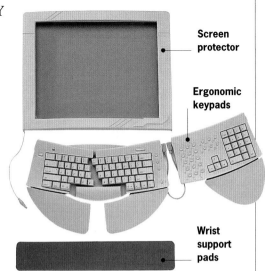

Screen protector

Ergonomic keypads

Wrist support pads

by the phosphorescent substance lining the tube itself. The amount of ultraviolet light emitted is small—far less than that received from sunlight.

COMPUTERS

The phenomenal growth of computers in all sectors of industry has been accompanied by growing concerns about health and safety problems associated with monitors, or visual display units. Working long hours at a monitor can produce a range of physical and psychological health problems. Some of the symptoms are relatively minor and disappear once the work is stopped, but they can, in combination with other factors, become worse if intense computer work is continued over a long period of time.

Many of the health problems attributed to monitors are actually the result of the poor design of the work area or the furniture that holds the unit or a lack of knowledge among people who do not use computers regularly. The current state of scientific knowledge and research on a great many of the problems allegedly associated with computer operation does not permit strong conclusions to be drawn. Nevertheless, it is possible to take precautions to lower risks and safeguard health.

The single most common health problem associated with computer monitors is eyestrain. This can result in blurred vision, fatigue, and soreness of the eyes. It can also cause an aching head, neck, or back. It is sometimes argued that long-term use of monitors can affect eyesight permanently,

but there is little medical evidence to support such claims. What is clear, however, is that people with uncorrected or imperfectly corrected visual defects suffer greater eyestrain from using a monitor than those with properly corrected vision. Because eye defects become worse with age, this is a problem that increasingly affects older workers.

There have been reports in many countries of an increase in repetitive stress injuries of the fingers, hands, wrists, and arms, such as tenosynovitis and carpal tunnel syndrome (see page 124). These occur most often among data-entry and word-processing personnel, who enter material into computer systems at high speeds for long hours. Any worker suffering from chronic soreness or tenderness in any part of the hands or arms should seek medical advice. (One test for carpal tunnel syndrome is to hold the backs of the hands together with the wrists fully flexed for one minute. If you feel numbness, tingling, or pain, you may have the condition.)

There has been widespread concern about the effects that monitors may have on pregnant women, and a possible link between high rates of miscarriages in those who use computers regularly. However there is no conclusive evidence that such a link exists. The most commonly suggested cause of these problems has been radiation, but the only measurable levels of radiation have been in bands of very low frequency or extra-low frequency, and exposures to these levels have not been found to cause biological changes in human beings.

Chamomile tea tonic
A tonic made from chamomile tea can help to revive tired or overstrained eyes. Mix 30 ml (2 tbsp) cooled chamomile tea with 30 ml (2 tbsp) witch hazel. Add 1 tsp castor oil and 2 drops of frankincense essential oil. Combine well. Dip cotton balls into the tonic, squeeze out the excess liquid, and place the balls over your closed eyelids.

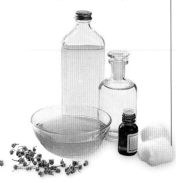

Indoor Plants

Bringing plants into your workplace is one way to brighten up the room and make it visually more attractive. If you choose the right plants and care for them well, they can also help make your work environment healthier.

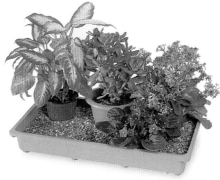

CREATING HUMIDITY
Many plants need to grow in a humid atmosphere. To create extra humidity for them, place the pots in a tray half filled with small pebbles or clay balls, then pour in a shallow layer of water.

Most people know that plants can improve air quality, but they may be less aware that some actually absorb airborne pollutants. Spider plant, philodendron, sansevieria, dracaena, and golden pothos are believed to absorb formaldehyde, a common indoor pollutant; dracaena and spathiphyllum may absorb benzene and trichloroethylene; spathiphyllum may also be effective in mopping up electrical radiation from televisions and computers. The moisture given off by plants not only humidifies the air but also appears to suppress airborne microbes. And a study at Washington State University showed that people with plants in their offices were 12 percent more productive and had lower blood pressure.

People who are allergic to molds may have trouble with indoor plants. Putting a layer of pebbles over the soil seems to help prevent this.

CARING FOR OFFICE PLANTS

Plants around the office can improve the atmosphere by adding a touch of color and life. However, an office filled with dying or unhealthy plants does not, for obvious reasons, provide any benefits. Feng shui experts believe that dead plants can in fact create unhealthy chi and sap the energy that is flowing around them, while healthy, vigorous plants are thought to balance electrical radiation, bringing their own natural energy to the work environment. To ensure that your office plants remain as healthy and effective as possible, follow the simple steps given below.

▶ *Take note of watering instructions that come with the plant and follow them; too much water can be as bad as too little.*

▶ *Make sure the soil is damp but not soaking wet. This helps plants to create a humid atmosphere.*

▶ *Indoor plants often like being grouped together; they create a mini climate for themselves that helps keep them healthy.*

▶ *Do not move plants around too much. If they seem to be happy in one place, leave them there.*

▶ *Regularly remove any faded or dead flowers and damaged or dried leaves. This will encourage new growth.*

▶ *Be sure to feed your plants regularly during the spring and summer growing seasons.*

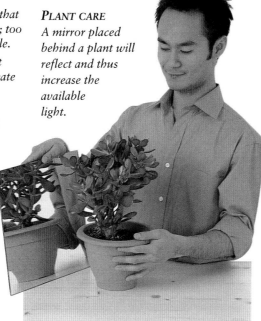

PLANT CARE
A mirror placed behind a plant will reflect and thus increase the available light.

THE IMPORTANCE OF HUMIDITY

Many plants require an indoor atmosphere that is fairly moist in order to thrive; humidity of about 60 percent is considered ideal. However, the level of humidity in an average, centrally heated office or home is usually 20 to 50 percent. It is healthier for you to have a more humid environment as well, so in winter place bowls of water in front of heaters (these will release water vapor into the air) and/or turn off the central heating for a while.

One rare potential problem with monitor use is photosensitive epilepsy. Approximately 0.5 percent of the population have epilepsy, and of those, up to 3 percent have a sensitivity to flickering lights or certain light patterns. The condition is more common among children than adults. Most people who have this sensitivity will know of their condition from watching television, which flickers like a monitor. If you suspect that you may suffer from photosensitive epilepsy, you should consult your doctor before working on a computer.

STRESS AT WORK

Stress at work can be damaging to physical and mental health, and it is not restricted to the archetypal high-flying executive who works long hours. Low-paid workers are often in jobs with little security and few benefits, such as health insurance, pension, and sick pay, which can also cause stress. In addition, some people may be facing stress at home that is caused by poor housing or limited educational opportunities. In particular, women who have little education often have no alternative but to take low-paying or part-time jobs, which can be the cause of considerable personal stress.

Although *stress* is a commonly used term, it is difficult to define. Everyone is subject to stress, yet our understanding of it is far from complete. The term *stress* can be used to describe a number of things, including distress, fatigue, and a feeling of not being able to cope, but it is also a driving force that can push people to work more vigorously and effectively. Individuals respond to situations in different ways. For example, some find a repetitive job comfortable, whereas others find it frustrating and therefore stressful because it provides no challenge. Similarly, some persons are able to manage a stressful working situation for a long period of time, while others quickly find it intolerable.

It is possible to measure physical causes of stress, such as noise and temperature levels, but it is more difficult to measure the effect of a heavy workload or conflict. Stress will eventually result if the demands placed on you outstrip your resources to cope with them or if there is insufficient time to complete a task properly.

The body itself has a built-in mechanism designed to deal with a dangerous situation. Known as the "fight or flight" response, this

continued on page 132

ARE YOU SITTING COMFORTABLY?

A good chair can help you avoid back, shoulder, and neck pain. When seated in your office chair, you should be able to sit comfortably with your feet flat on the floor. Depending on your height, the seat should be 17 to 19 inches from the floor. There are many kinds of special back-support chairs on the market, as well as a number of seating accessories that can help to prevent or relieve back pain.

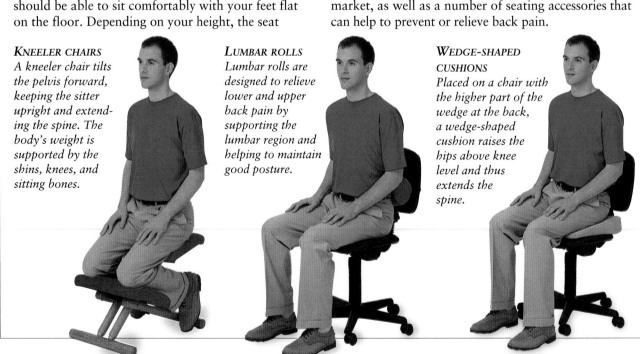

KNEELER CHAIRS
A kneeler chair tilts the pelvis forward, keeping the sitter upright and extending the spine. The body's weight is supported by the shins, knees, and sitting bones.

LUMBAR ROLLS
Lumbar rolls are designed to relieve lower and upper back pain by supporting the lumbar region and helping to maintain good posture.

WEDGE-SHAPED CUSHIONS
Placed on a chair with the higher part of the wedge at the back, a wedge-shaped cushion raises the hips above knee level and thus extends the spine.

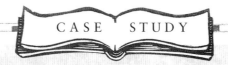
A Harassed Manager

While many employers like open-plan offices, believing they improve communication and raise productivity, for some workers they can prove to be a very difficult environment in which to work. Constant distractions and interruptions can make it hard to complete jobs that demand a great deal of concentration, and the result may be increased stress.

Vicky is a 35-year-old word processor who has recently been promoted to manager of her team. Although she is used to working hard and has plenty of experience dealing with the problems faced by her staff, she is becoming increasingly stressed and feels unable to cope. The office space is an open plan, and there are no partitions or private areas where she can deal with confidential concerns or shut herself off to concentrate properly on more difficult tasks. She feels increasingly unable to prioritize her work, and constant interruptions mean that she is falling behind. Her sleep at night is suffering, and she has lost her appetite. In desperation she has arranged to see her doctor to ask for sleeping pills.

WHAT SHOULD VICKY DO?

Vicky needs a thorough checkup with her primary care doctor to be certain there is no physical cause for her insomnia and loss of appetite. She also has to look at how stress at work is affecting her health. She should talk to her boss about the fact that the layout of the office is making her feel that she has insufficient control over her work and seek advice on ways to improve the working environment. Vicky also needs to talk to her colleagues about the difficulties she is having and enlist their support for change. It is very important that she keep her work in perspective and allow time in her life for proper rest and relaxation. A form of de-stressing exercise, such as t'ai chi, may help.

Action Plan

WORK
Take time to organize the day and include periods for quiet concentration. Discuss concerns and solutions with boss and set clear guidelines for staff.

STRESS
Deal with work problems as they arise. Take up a physical activity to counter the effects of stress. Try to relax in the evening.

EMOTIONAL HEALTH
Talk over concerns with staff to increase confidence in own ability to cope. Allow sufficient time to complete jobs properly.

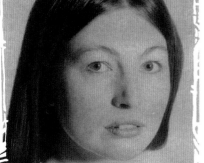

WORK
A lack of privacy and an inability to concentrate on work can lead to job dissatisfaction.

EMOTIONAL HEALTH
Feelings of insecurity and worries about work performance can create a vicious cycle of anxiety.

STRESS
Not being able to complete tasks properly can cause stress to develop and lead to physical symptoms that disrupt your life.

HOW THINGS TURNED OUT FOR VICKY

Vicky's boss arranged for low partitions to be erected in the office to provide some privacy while still allowing easy communication. Vicky talked to her staff about this new arrangement and explained how she needed a couple of uninterrupted hours each day. She began exercising at lunchtime, which helped her to relax and burn off some stress. Within a month Vicky felt in control and was sleeping and eating much better.

The Karate Teacher

People tend to see karate as an aggressive sport with little to offer the general public. In fact, it is an excellent form of exercise for relieving stress, while also being a very useful form of self-defense for both men and women.

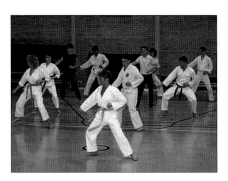

KARATE EQUIPMENT
The main equipment for karate is a suit called karategi, *or* gi, *which should be a size too large to allow ease of movement. Fist mitts, shin guards, and groin protectors are also useful during practice.*

Karate is a martial art of unarmed combat that has strong philosophical undertones. Although it is based on ancient Chinese forms of boxing, it first developed in Okinawa (where weapons were once banned) and then moved to mainland Japan, where it evolved into the traditional form known today. Its purpose is to put you in full control of the muscular power of your body so it can be used with force and accuracy at any instant.

Traditional karate was developed with the principal aim of defeating one's own fear and anger rather than fighting an opponent. The sport is therefore as much a form of mental and emotional training as it is physical, with the emphasis on developing concentration, discipline, serenity, and self-respect.

What are the different styles of karate?
There are four main schools of karate. The basic techniques are common to each school, but there are differences in the way they are practiced. *Shotokan* is the most popular style. It uses low, strong stances, and the emphasis is on generating maximum power. *Goju ryu* is very traditional, and competition is not particularly important. It incorporates a fitness program designed to increase strength. *Shito ryu* incorporates characteristics of both Shotokan and Goju ryu, and competition is very important in this school of karate. *Wado ryu* avoids direct confrontation of force against force and instead relies much more on sophisticated evasion movements.

How do I find an instructor?
Most karate instructors teach in a club, and if they are members of the U.S. Martial Arts Association, they have had to pass recognized grading requirements. An instructor must hold at least a black belt, the highest level of karate achievement, and most have one and usually several degrees added to the black belt.

THE KNIFE BLOCK
In this basic karate move, a combatant catches the forearm of his opponent and attacks his opponent's ribs with the other hand.

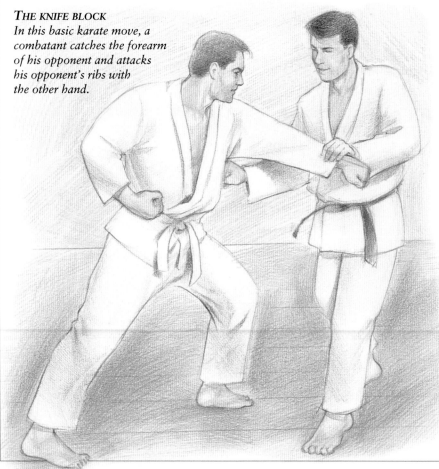

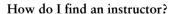

Origins

Karate dates from the 17th century but in its modern form was developed in the 20th century in Japan. Its name, adopted in the 1930s, means literally "empty hand." The most popular style, called Shotokan, comes from Okinawa.

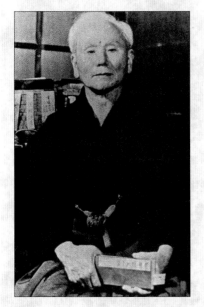

FOUNDING FATHER
Ghichin Funakoshi developed Shotokan karate to help students generate maximum power.

How fit do I need to be?

Karate is a reasonably strenuous form of exercise that requires a fair degree of flexibility. It is sensible to consult your doctor before you take up the sport, especially if you are a novice over the age of 40. Whatever your fitness level when you start, however, it will be greatly improved after just a few months.

You should inform your instructor if you suffer from any condition that might affect your training. The instructor can keep an eye on your performance and perhaps spot any dangerous symptoms before you do.

If you have a cold, avoid any sharp blows to the chest and sudden training spurts because both of these can have serious side effects on the heart muscle.

What clothing should I wear?

As a beginner it is fine to wear a T-shirt and track suit pants, but if you intend to continue with karate, you will need a suit called a *karategi*, or *gi* for short. You should buy your suit too large because you will need plenty of room in the thigh and groin areas to allow you to lift your knee up without hindrance.

Karate is performed in bare feet, but you should wear a pair of flip-flops to keep your feet clean as you walk between the changing rooms and the training hall.

What happens in a training session?

Respect for your instructor and classmates is very important in karate; even the training hall, or *dojo*, is treated with respect. You are expected to bow upon entering and leaving the dojo and to maintain a calm and well-behaved demeanor at all times during the training session. The class is first called to order with the students lined up according to their proficiency; the person in front of you should be wearing the same color belt as you are. The class begins and ends with everyone kneeling and bowing to the teacher, or *sensei*, and to classmates.

The teacher's role in a session is to guide the students not only in the correct way to perform movements but also in the underlying principles and philosophy of the sport.

What are katas?

Katas are training drills that teach the basic principles of techniques and their application, plus focus, endurance, speed, and balance. Initially you will practice a kata in individual steps, according to the instructor's command. Later, you will perform them in a particular sequence with the aim of achieving both fluidity and balance. Each sequence consists of a series of techniques separated by pauses and represents a response to an imaginary sparring situation.

WHAT YOU CAN DO AT HOME

As with all types of exercise, it is essential to warm up your body thoroughly before beginning training. Karate works parts of your body that are not used often, so it is especially important to carry out a warm-up that is appropriate for karate training to prevent any aches, pains, or injury.

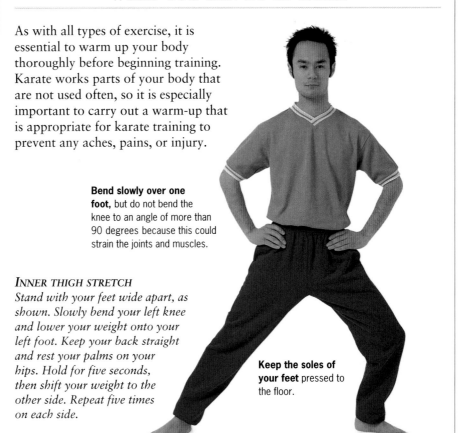

Bend slowly over one foot, but do not bend the knee to an angle of more than 90 degrees because this could strain the joints and muscles.

INNER THIGH STRETCH
Stand with your feet wide apart, as shown. Slowly bend your left knee and lower your weight onto your left foot. Keep your back straight and rest your palms on your hips. Hold for five seconds, then shift your weight to the other side. Repeat five times on each side.

Keep the soles of your feet pressed to the floor.

reaction is useful in many situations, such as the physical threat of an attack or accident. Stress can be beneficial in other ways too, helping someone to meet a work deadline or win a race. When the body responds to stress, the heart rate increases, muscles tighten up, and blood sugar levels rise as more fats are ejected into the blood in preparation for a spurt of physical activity. If these responses are repeated continuously and not burned off by physical activity, they can be harmful.

Stress also triggers the release of hormones that are needed for increased activity, but they can cause damage in excess amounts. The links between adrenaline and coronary heart disease are well known. In the short term adrenaline helps the body to react quickly, but too much over an extended period has an adverse effect on the brain and makes a person feel very tired.

The symptoms of chronic stress are wide-ranging. They can include constant indecision, loss of appetite, unexplained weight loss, headache, backache, rash, and difficulty in sleeping. If some of these symptoms persist over a long period, they may eventually lead to other health problems, such as hypertension or heart disease.

Like any other occupational hazard, stress needs to be tackled at its source. Because it can arise from a variety of factors and there is no common danger level, everyone must be aware of stress factors in the workplace and do their best to control them, both in the environment and in themselves.

VIOLENCE AT WORK

In some jobs, such as police work or military service, a certain level of violence is expected as an occupational hazard. However, violence in the workplace is now far more widespread and not limited to such specific occupations. Public transportation employees are at risk on buses, trains, and subways. A substantial number of incidents are occurring in the health services and to a lesser extent in the retail industry. Other workers at risk include public personnel at government agencies, and lately even teachers have been under attack.

While employers cannot be expected to solve the underlying problems of violence in society, it is clear that there is a substantial amount that they can do to reduce the risk of violence to their employees. It is because the problem of violence is often associated with the main purpose of an organization—providing a service to the public—that the task of prevention or control is seen as an integral part of the management of a business.

Defining what is meant by violence is an essential but surprisingly difficult task for anyone involved in trying to investigate

A HEALTHY WORKPLACE
Every occupation carries certain health risks. By observing some simple precautions, you can avoid most accidents and injuries.

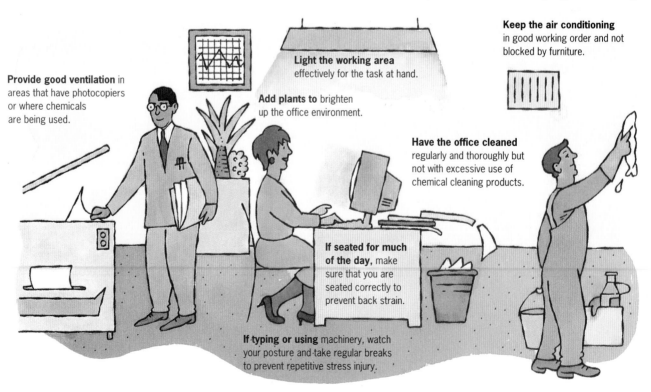

Provide good ventilation in areas that have photocopiers or where chemicals are being used.

Light the working area effectively for the task at hand.

Add plants to brighten up the office environment.

Keep the air conditioning in good working order and not blocked by furniture.

Have the office cleaned regularly and thoroughly but not with excessive use of chemical cleaning products.

If seated for much of the day, make sure that you are seated correctly to prevent back strain.

If typing or using machinery, watch your posture and take regular breaks to prevent repetitive stress injury.

manage, or prevent it at work. Clearly the definition must include incidents that cause death or injury, whether serious or minor, but threats, whether or not with a weapon, are also an issue, even if no injury actually occurs. Constant verbal abuse is another factor; it can actually damage health because it is a major source of stress. Sometimes violence is not limited to the workplace but follows workers to their homes or takes the form of attacks on their property.

Employers are clearly under an obligation to recognize the potential of workplace violence and take measures to control it. In a famous case a store clerk successfully sued her employer after the store she worked in was robbed for the second time because the managers had ignored the precautionary measures she had suggested be taken after the first incident.

People are sometimes reluctant to report a violent incident for reasons that relate directly to the way their work is organized. Some fear the incident could be seen as their own failure—their mishandling of a situation. Some do not want the attention that a report would bring them and, if there is an absence of counseling or support for victims, may see no point in reporting violence. And there is still a macho atmosphere in many workplaces, where the "I can handle anything" attitude is common.

Workers must be encouraged to report threatening incidents and be assured that their employer will deal with the issue. For most people risk is more likely to arise because of several factors coming together rather than a single cause. Examples include handling money in an isolated situation, operating a bus at the end of the day, and coping with angry and distressed patients and relatives in an emergency room at night (see checklist, page 134).

The risk of violence is an occupational hazard that must be tackled in a systematic way. The first step must be to discover where and why there is a risk. This will very often be different in each occupation and specific function. Without this type of investigation, any preventive measures are likely to be ineffective. The success of any measure can be assessed only by its relevance to any one situation where violence is a possible outcome.

The question of violence should be taken into account when decisions are being made about the design or alteration of buildings; when staffing levels, working practices, communication channels, and procedures are being established; or when training needs are assessed. These decisions should not be left solely to management but should include professionals who specialize in dealing with security and safety.

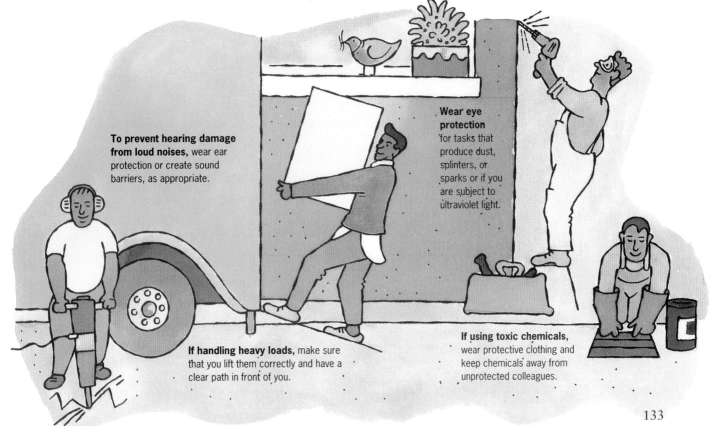

To prevent hearing damage from loud noises, wear ear protection or create sound barriers, as appropriate.

Wear eye protection for tasks that produce dust, splinters, or sparks or if you are subject to ultraviolet light.

If handling heavy loads, make sure that you lift them correctly and have a clear path in front of you.

If using toxic chemicals, wear protective clothing and keep chemicals away from unprotected colleagues.

LIFTING AND CARRYING

About a quarter of all accidents reported every year are connected with the handling of heavy loads. These incidents cost a great deal in money and human suffering. Lifting a load incorrectly or lifting one that is too heavy can cause damage to the back muscles or spine. Such injuries can literally disable you, making physical activity either impossible or extremely painful. Back injuries can rarely be seen in X-rays and can be difficult to treat. Rest is usually the only cure, but back injuries are often slow to heal, and once damage is done, the injury can easily recur.

Accidents that happen when handling heavy loads can also cause strains and sprains in other parts of the body and can even lead to further accidents. For example, losing control of a heavy or dangerous load can endanger others.

Back injuries on the job are not limited to the traditional industries like freight loading. Nurses suffer a disproportionate number of back injuries as a result of lifting patients, which is an unavoidable part of their work. Many sectors of industry and commerce require some degree of manual handling, so it is a concern of which employees should be aware.

There are four principal approaches to reducing the hazards of manual handling: eliminating the problem by using mechanical lifting or automated procedures; altering the way manual handling work is organized to reduce its scale; adapting tasks so that manual handling is reduced; and training people properly for the work.

The solution to manual handling problems in the workplace often involves a mixture of all these approaches. But tackling such problems is rarely a one-time exercise. It requires a sustained campaign, with

CHECKLIST
Some jobs are riskier than others when it comes to potential violence. People whose work involves any of the following should take extra precautions.

- ✔ *Handling money*
- ✔ *Providing care, advice, or information*
- ✔ *Working with violent people*
- ✔ *Dealing with complaints*
- ✔ *Having the power to act against the public in an enforcement situation*
- ✔ *Working alone*
- ✔ *Working odd hours*
- ✔ *Being isolated geographically from other employees*
- ✔ *Working in the community*
- ✔ *Working in badly lit areas*
- ✔ *Not working on the employer's premises*
- ✔ *Working on multi-occupation premises*

short-, medium-, and long-term goals. There is no such thing as a safe maximum weight that can be lifted. Although weight is an important factor, it is only one element that needs to be considered in deciding how much force is needed to move a given load under specific conditions.

People vary greatly in their ability to handle loads safely. What may be safe for the majority of persons in a given situation may still leave a minority at risk. Task conditions can make a big difference also. Another way of looking at the problem is to consider the amount of overall manual handling to which an individual is subjected. Handling moderate-sized loads frequently can pose as great a risk as handling heavy loads only occasionally. This is because the effects of repeated lifting and pushing on muscles, joints, and ligaments tend to be cumulative. For instance, a report on the handling of patients in health care establishments estimated that nurses were moving the equivalent of about 2,750 pounds an hour. Lifting tasks can be eased by using mechanical lifting devices whenever feasible and training all employees correctly for their jobs.

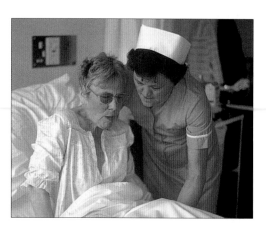

NURSING INJURIES
Nurses and other caregivers are subject to a variety of back injuries and strains because of lifting patients from or into their beds. Mechanical lifting devices can help with the problem, but these are not always convenient. Proper training in lifting techniques is essential.

CHAPTER 6

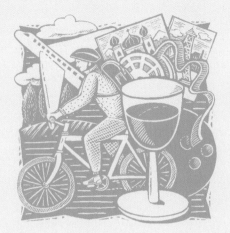

OUT AND ABOUT

---

*The leisure and entertainment industries
are booming as the amount we spend on dining
out, weekend excursions, and vacation travel
continues to rise. To ensure that such activities
remain the pleasurable and enriching experiences
they are meant to be, we must be aware of
potential health risks and take steps to protect
ourselves and those around us as well.*

PLACES TO DINE, DRINK, AND DANCE

A good night out can do you a world of good, but are you getting more than you ordered in a bar or restaurant? And what is the leisure industry doing to protect its customers?

As leisure time has increased and disposable income has grown, Western society has developed a growing taste for recreation and entertainment. Social activities and leisure pursuits can contribute positively to health and well-being, but it is important to realize that the places where they occur can have an impact on health.

SMOKING

Tobacco smoke is one of the main threats to health in public places, especially in places for socializing, such as bars, restaurants, and clubs. Passive, or environmental, smoking is now recognized as a major risk factor for people who themselves do not normally smoke. Recent studies show that nonsmokers who breathe in second-hand tobacco smoke throughout their lives increase their risk of contracting lung cancer and heart disease by 10 to 30 percent. In the majority of enclosed public places, such as buses and trains, movie theaters, and concert halls, smoking has been banned to create a smoke-free environment. Throughout this country smoking is now banned completely

in many office buildings and restaurants as well, but this trend has not yet become widespread elsewhere in the world.

An increasing number of restaurant owners are recognizing, however, that popular consensus demands that at least a section of the eating area be devoted to nonsmokers. But because of the internal arrangements of many premises, this is often little more than a gesture toward political correctness because tobacco smoke still wafts through the overall space. If a nonsmoking area is truly to work, good ventilation or air conditioning is required to ensure that smoke stays well away from the nonsmoking areas of the room.

Because of growing support for the view that smoking and eating should not mix, smoke-free restaurants can be found in many areas. Smoke-free bars are less common. The culture of public houses involves a strong correlation between smoking and drinking, which makes this a far more intractable problem. Some cities have passed ordinances against smoking in bars, but enforcing the regulation is difficult and needs corresponding social pressure.

Good ventilation is the key to enabling customers to enjoy a social drink in a relatively smoke-free atmosphere. However, this is often hard to achieve because ventilation that is strong enough to keep smoke limited to certain areas inevitably creates strong air currents or drafts that some persons may find uncomfortable.

On January 1, 1998, smoking was banned in all bars in California. The law was prompted by the high incidence of lung cancer and other smoking-related illnesses among bartenders and waiters. The ban has faced considerable opposition from many

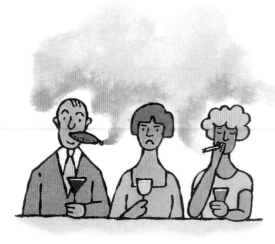

PASSIVE SMOKING
Inhaling other people's tobacco smoke in bars and restaurants is not only unpleasant but also dangerous. Medical research has shown that nonsmokers exposed to smoke on a regular basis have a higher risk of developing lung cancer and heart disease than those who are not regularly exposed.

THE STORY OF *E. COLI*

In November 1996, one of the world's worst recorded outbreaks of *Escherichia coli* occurred in Wishaw, Lanarkshire, in Scotland. Twenty-one people died and some 160 were admitted to a hospital. Cold and cooked meats from a local butcher were blamed for the outbreak.

Only thorough cooking kills *E. coli*. The bacterium has become known as the hamburger bug because it is common in ground beef (grinding spreads the germ throughout the meat). *E. coli* invades the human intestine and multiplies rapidly, causing widespread inflammation of the gut, symptoms of which include abdominal cramps, diarrhea, vomiting, and a low-grade fever. Most at risk are the elderly and young children.

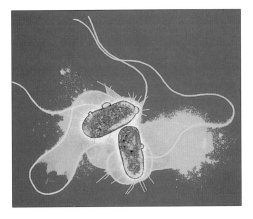

DEADLY BACTERIA
E. coli *is a rod-shaped bacterium found in the intestinal tract of animals. It clings to the surface of meats and lurks in unpasteurized milk and multiplies rapidly at room temperature.*

smokers, and it remains to be seen whether it will be successful. Because of the rising health costs for tobacco-related illnesses, however, pressure to eliminate smoking in our society will probably continue.

RESTAURANTS

Hygiene standards are very important in places where food is sold or consumed. Reported cases of food poisoning are on the increase, and infection by some organisms, such as salmonella and *E. coli,* can be fatal

Food handling practices must be scrupulous to ensure that no cross contamination occurs between raw and cooked foods. The kitchen area and all appliances must be kept clean and in good working order, and all employees working in the kitchen or serving the food must be trained in the rules of basic food hygiene. If you are eating in a restaurant and are served something that looks undercooked or has an off taste, send it back to the kitchen. You are perfectly within your rights to do so. Regulations for restaurants and other food establishments are enforced by local health departments, and you can report infractions to them.

NIGHTCLUBS

A number of issues specific to nightclubs need to be enforced for everyone to enjoy a night out without risk. Overcrowding can be especially dangerous. The maximum number of people allowed in a club or disco at one time is set by the appropriate licensing authority and is normally based on information from the local fire department. The purpose of setting a maximum occupancy number is to ensure that the means of escape in the event of a fire is adequate for the number of people on the premises. This means that exact numbers must be recorded and controlled at the entrance. Emergency exits should be unlocked during occupancy, clearly marked, and free of obstructions.

The noise level in clubs is another hazard, but one that is very difficult to control. In most communities there is no official legal limit on the noise volumes that the public can be exposed to in nightclubs or bars, but some legislation does apply now to people who are employed within a club (although

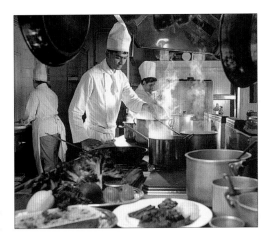

HYGIENE STANDARDS
Food poisoning is on the increase. It is very important that any establishment where food is prepared and/or consumed adhere to strict hygiene rules. The kitchen should always be kept scrupulously clean. Chefs and other kitchen employees should wear clean clothing and aprons and hats that cover their hair.

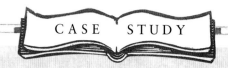
A Tinnitus Sufferer

Loud noise can often bring on tinnitus, or ringing in the ears, and young people who listen to loud rock music are at particular risk for developing it. In some people the complaint may just be irritating, but in others it can lead to sleepless nights and stress. Taking some simple precautions can help to prevent more serious long-term damage.

John is a 19-year-old auto mechanic who goes to a local nightclub every Friday and Saturday night and has also begun working there as a disc jockey on two week-nights. He tends to skip breakfast, especially if he has been working at the club the night before, because he gets home late and stays in bed as long as possible the next morning.

Although he enjoys both of his jobs, John is feeling permanently tired, but more worrisome is the onset of a low ringing sound in his ears that sometimes prevents him from sleeping. His doctor has told him that his ears have been damaged by constant exposure to loud noise and that the problem could be permanent. The diagnosis has made John very depressed.

WHAT SHOULD JOHN DO?

John must stop exposing his ears to constant loud noise to keep the problem from getting worse. When he is at the club or using noisy machinery at the garage, he should wear earplugs or, better yet, ear-muffs, to protect his ears from further damage. He can try playing soft music or a white sound machine at night to mask the ringing and help him get to sleep.

John's doctor also told him that he must improve his lifestyle by getting enough rest and eating better. Although he is not suffering the effects of his neglect now, he may in the future. John should make sure that he eats regular, well-balanced meals, especially breakfast, and that he takes time for exercise.

Action Plan

WORK
Cut back on evening work or try to arrange for more flexible working hours during the day to allow time for more rest and relaxation.

DIET
Eat regular meals. Prepare more food at home and eat fresh food rather than take-out and frozen foods. Make an effort to have a good breakfast every day.

HEALTH
Avoid loud noise as much as possible and wear earmuffs or earplugs in noisy surroundings.

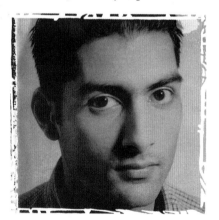

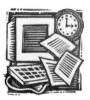

WORK
Physically stressful work can cause fatigue and depression, while very high noise levels can damage hearing.

DIET
A poor diet can exacerbate existing emotional and physical health problems.

HEALTH
Not taking care of your health can cause chronic problems later on in life.

HOW THINGS TURNED OUT FOR JOHN

John negotiated with his employer to come in later on the mornings after he has been working at the club, and he cut down on the time he spends at the club on weekends. He wears ear protection at the garage and when he is out clubbing, and he is now eating more freshly prepared meals and fruit rather than fast food. Although he still has tinnitus, John is more relaxed about it and finds that as long as he is not overtired, he can cope.

this is notoriously difficult to enforce). From a health point of view, it is undesirable for continuous noise levels to exceed 95 decibels (db) or for the peak noise level to exceed 140 db. And loudspeakers should be located at least 10 feet from the audience.

Prolonged exposure to high levels of noise can result in temporary hearing loss, tinnitus, or permanent hearing loss (see page 63). If you are exposed to high levels of noise at work, you must be extra careful to limit noise levels in your social and leisure time. Take earplugs to a club or rock concert; you will still be able to hear the music but will protect your ears from further damage.

The special lighting effects that are a feature of many modern nightclubs also pose potential problems. Display lasers, if not set up and managed correctly, can be very dangerous because they rely on the human blink

response to ensure that there is no eye damage. You should be aware that alcohol and drugs may affect this reaction and never look directly into a display laser because this could damage your sight.

Strobe lights can present risks to epileptics. If such lights are used, the club should give adequate warning at the entrance. Although flicker-sensitive epilepsy is rare, it is easily triggered, and there is a high risk that people with the condition will experience a full epileptic seizure. Flicker rates of strobe lights should be kept at or below four flashes per second if possible, because only 5 percent of the flicker-sensitive population is at risk of an attack at this level.

Ultraviolet light is a common component of a nightclub lighting rig. These lights should be well maintained to restrict exposure to UVB radiation.

The dangers of dehydration

Drink plenty of water when you are out dancing. Vigorous exercise like dancing, especially when mixed with alcohol consumption, can cause dehydration, characterized by headache, exhaustion, and dizziness. It is advisable to drink water regularly throughout the evening.

DEALING WITH AN EPILEPTIC SEIZURE

Epileptic seizures can be very traumatic, and there is only a brief warning period for them. Basic first aid is essential if you are with someone who is experiencing a seizure. Never restrain or lift the person unless he or she is in danger of further injury. Loosen any tight clothing around the neck and protect the head. Once the seizure ends, place the patient in the recovery position (see below). This position is used for many

conditions that require first aid because it ensures that the person can breathe freely but still allows fluids, such as vomit or blood, to drain away to prevent choking. It also promotes good circulation and keeps the body in a comfortable and stable position until medical help arrives. The position should not be used, however, if the person is not breathing or if there is a possibility of a spinal, neck, or other serious injury.

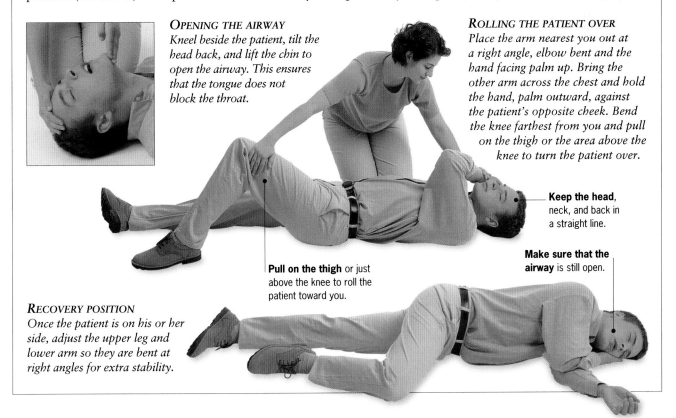

OPENING THE AIRWAY
Kneel beside the patient, tilt the head back, and lift the chin to open the airway. This ensures that the tongue does not block the throat.

ROLLING THE PATIENT OVER
Place the arm nearest you out at a right angle, elbow bent and the hand facing palm up. Bring the other arm across the chest and hold the hand, palm outward, against the patient's opposite cheek. Bend the knee farthest from you and pull on the thigh or the area above the knee to turn the patient over.

Keep the head, neck, and back in a straight line.

Make sure that the airway is still open.

Pull on the thigh or just above the knee to roll the patient toward you.

RECOVERY POSITION
Once the patient is on his or her side, adjust the upper leg and lower arm so they are bent at right angles for extra stability.

SAFETY IN YOUR CAR

The rise of the car in the 20th century was one of the biggest changes that happened to the the world. And using a car safely has been one of the biggest challenges.

The automobile has changed life dramatically since the 19th century. In 1890, 80 percent of journeys undertaken were on foot or by bicycle; in 1990 these two ways of getting around represented less than 3 percent. Although the car has had a positive impact in many ways, it has also had negative effects on the environment and health, which some people feel now outweigh its benefits. Car occupants make up 62 percent of all road casualties.

Over the past few decades, vehicle engineering and design have greatly improved to better protect both drivers and passengers. Many features, including more effective brakes, are intended to reduce the likelihood of accidents, while others, such as air bags, are designed to reduce the severity of injuries if one should occur.

In order to benefit fully from the safety features of an automobile, the driver should sit in the correct position, with the seat positioned so that the clutch and/or brake can be easily depressed while the knee is slightly bent but without the knee touching the dashboard or steering wheel. The seat back should be at an angle to give support while enabling the driver to hold the wheel with elbows slightly bent. Both hands should be on the wheel in the recommended positions of 10 o'clock and 2 o'clock.

SAFETY FEATURES

The main protection system in cars is, of course, the seat belt, which is intended to prevent automobile occupants from being thrown about inside the vehicle or from being ejected through a door or the front windshield in an accident.

Since fitting cars with seat belts became compulsory, it is known that the belts have saved thousands of lives and prevented tens of thousands of serious injuries. Most states now mandate the use of seat belts at least for front-seat occupants, and all 50 states and U.S. territories have laws covering the use of child restraints, but the laws vary in content and enforcement.

To be effective, seat belts must be worn as snugly as possible. The lap belt should rest across the pelvic region or the top of the thighs, not across the stomach. The diagonal belt should cross the chest and shoulder, not go under the arm or over the neck.

Child restraints

Seat belts are designed for adults and are not suitable for children under a certain height and weight. Child safety seats and belts can prevent injuries and save lives, but they must be suitable for the height and weight of the child (see box, opposite page) and be used and installed correctly. You should follow the instructions carefully, and if you have a problem, ask the store to install the restraint for you or show you how to do it correctly. Properly installed devices reduce the risk of death by 71 percent for infants and by 54 percent for children ages 1 to 4.

SAFETY FEATURES
Safety features are rigorously tested by auto manufacturers using dummies to simulate what happens to passengers. Despite this, only after their introduction was it discovered that air bags can increase the risk of serious injury for some people—especially children in the front passenger seat and drivers who are short and therefore position their seat close to the steering wheel. Some cars now have a switch to turn the air bag off for people who are at risk.

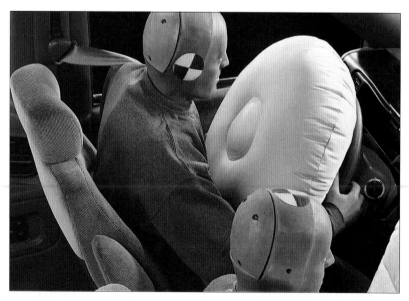

CAR SEATS FOR CHILD SAFETY

When buying a child restraint, it is very important to choose the right one. Ask the staff at the store to show you how to install it in the car correctly. Always buy a new restraint; secondhand ones have often lost much of their strength and may no longer meet regulations. Take your child along when choosing a new seat to judge which kind is suitable and is the right size.

CHILD RESTRAINTS
The various types of seat belts and car seats available for children are designed for maximum safety according to the weight and height of the child.

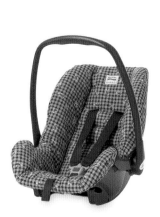

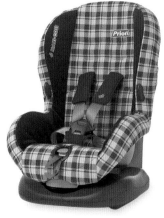

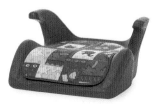

An infant seat with restraining strap is used from birth to 12 months, usually up to 22 pounds.

A forward-facing child seat is used from 1 to 4 years, or from about 22 to 40 pounds.

A securable booster cushion is used from 4 to 11 years, or from about 40 to 80 pounds.

Adult safety belts do not adequately protect all children between ages 4 and 12 (about 40 to 80 pounds). Car booster seats are the best way to protect them, but only about 5 percent of children are now provided with them. A child should never sit on an unsecured booster cushion or a regular cushion in the car because it could slip out from beneath the child in a collision, possibly resulting in more serious injury.

A baby up to 1 year old, or 22 pounds, should be placed in a rear-facing child safety seat and never in the front passenger seat of a vehicle that has a passenger air bag. (In fact, all children under age 12 are safer in the back seat. A number have been seriously injured or killed by an air bag.) After age 1 a child can be placed in a forward-facing seat because by that time the bones are hardening and the head and neck are less vulnerable.

Air bags

The majority of new cars are now fitted with air bags to supplement the protection provided by seat belts, and most models have them for both the driver and front passenger seats. An air bag inflates rapidly out of the steering wheel, dashboard, or door (in the case of a side-impact bag) and then immediately deflates, thus preventing a passenger from making violent contact with the steering wheel or dashboard in an accident. An air bag expands quickly in order to be fully inflated by the time a person's body moves in reaction to a crash. It is fully inflated within 50 milliseconds, which means it expands at up to 200 mph. Evidence suggests that thousands of lives have been saved by air bags. But there is concern that in some accidents air bags may actually have caused injuries as they inflated. (This is a greater problem in the United States than in Europe because American air bags are more powerful and larger than European ones.)

Since 1998 buyers have had the option of requesting an on/off switch for one or both air bags. It is granted if a child under age 12 must be placed in the front passenger seat, if a driver cannot keep 10 inches between the steering wheel and his or her breastbone, or if a passenger's fragile condition is more threatened by the impact of an air bag than by possible injury without it.

To maximize the protection offered by air bags and minimize any danger from them in an accident, always wear a seat belt and position your seat as far back from the dashboard or steering wheel as is safe and comfortable, making sure that you can easily reach all the controls and foot pedals.

SAFE TODDLERS
A front-facing child seat is recommended for children from the age of 1 to 4 years. It readily fits in the back seat of the car, provides all-round impact protection, and has a harness-style strap for extra security.

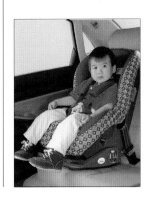

SAFE DRIVING TIPS

The number of automobiles and other vehicles on the road continues to climb, and vehicle accidents claim several thousand lives every year. Excess speed is often a factor and accounts for about 30 percent of all fatal crashes. Many more accidents result directly from loss of concentration or fatigue.

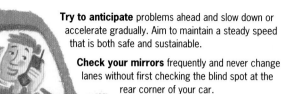

Try to anticipate problems ahead and slow down or accelerate gradually. Aim to maintain a steady speed that is both safe and sustainable.

Check your mirrors frequently and never change lanes without first checking the blind spot at the rear corner of your car.

Never use a cellular phone when driving; it prevents you from using both hands for driving and distracts your attention. A hands-free adapter is better, but calls are still distracting. The safest option is to pull off the road, then make your call.

Remain calm in all situations: aggression can cause accidents or lead to incidences of road rage.

When you need to read a map, stop well off the road. Attempting to read a map while driving is dangerous in two regards—it takes your hands off the wheel and your eyes off the road.

Keep your eyes on the road at all times and don't look at a passenger while talking.

Tune into a radio station or insert a cassette before you set off on your journey so you don't have to find a radio station or choose a cassette while driving.

Pull off the road to eat or drink. Doing so while driving is dangerous, and drinks can spill easily. Also, taking a break helps you maintain concentration.

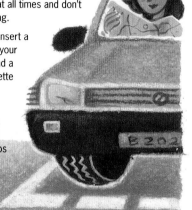

Head restraints

Commonly called headrests, the padded extensions at the top of car seats are actually restraints. They are designed to reduce whiplash injuries by preventing a person's head from being snapped back sharply in a collision. It is essential that your head restraint be properly positioned. Ideally, it should be about the width of two fingers away from the back of your head, not touching it. The top of the head restraint should be about level with your eyes so that support is provided for the neck in the event of an accident.

CONCENTRATION

Driving is a complex operation that requires 100 percent concentration the whole time. Any activity that distracts a person who is driving greatly increases the likelihood of an accident.

Many people feel that driving is wasted time, and they are tempted to do other things during a journey, such as using a cell phone, scribbling notes, applying makeup, scanning the radio stations, or reading a map. The latest research suggests that drivers look away from the road for about two seconds or more at frequent intervals when using a cellular phone. If you are traveling at 60 mph, this means that you will have traveled at least 88 feet without looking at the road. Even cell phones that have a hands-free adapter so the driver does not have to hold the instrument are dangerous because the conversation distracts the driver's attention from the road.

Smoking while driving can also distract you, especially when you are trying to find and light a cigarette or put one out. Furthermore, the carbon monoxide and other chemicals from cigarettes can affect your ability to concentrate.

Boredom can lead to accidents if your attention wanders, especially if you are driving a route you know very well or are on a long stretch of highway that is monotonous and hypnotic. Listening to music can help you to sustain attention levels—although some slow music can also have a hypnotic effect—but as a general rule, a driver should never engage in any other activity that detracts from his or her ability to safely navigate through traffic.

If at any time during a long journey you feel sleepy or start to lose your concentration, it is time to take a break at a roadside cafe or a specially designated rest stop. This will give you an opportunity to stretch your legs and get some fresh air, which will help you to stay alert until you reach your destination or take your next break.

TRANSPORTATION OPTIONS

Choosing transportation other than a car is one of the best things you can do to combat pollution, both globally and locally, and contribute to a healthier environment and personal lifestyle.

Most people would agree that using their car less and bicycling, walking, and/or riding public transportation more often would help to combat pollution. However, in many countries, especially those in the Western world, investments in new roads and ever better cars have far outstripped investments in public transportation and support for pedestrians and bicyclists. There is no doubt that many individuals love their cars and the feel-good factor associated with owning a certain model or color. The task of persuading them to leave their cars at home as much as possible is not an easy one.

Many people argue that their car gives them a level of comfort, privacy, and convenience not attainable on buses or trains. Nonetheless, government agencies, both national and local, have been working on initiatives to encourage walking and cycling and to make public transportation more convenient and attractive to people, and there are encouraging signs that these efforts are starting to pay off.

The first major government program to support public transportation was approved in 1964 with an act of Congress that established the Urban Mass Transit Authority in the Department of Transportation. Some

MODES OF TRANSPORTATION

The table below shows typical weekly use of various modes of transportation in the United Kingdom, averaged across the population in a 20-year period. Similar changes in ridership have occurred in many Western countries.

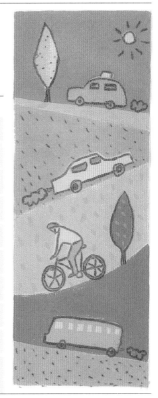

AVERAGE INDIVIDUAL USE OF TRANSPORTATION DURING A TYPICAL WEEK			
Transportation Method	**1975–76**	**1992–94**	**Percent Change**
Foot	1hr 32 min	1 hr 28 min	– 4 percent
Bicycle	8 min	6 min	– 25 percent
Motorcycle	2 min	1 min	– 50 percent
Car: driver	2 hr 38 min	3 hr 29 min	+ 52 percent
Car: passenger	1 hr 7 min	1 hr 33 min	+ 39 percent
Local bus	52 min	39 min	– 25 percent
Interurban bus	5 min	3 min	– 40 percent
Train	16 min	20 min	+ 25 percent
Taxi and other	8 min	13 min	+ 63 percent

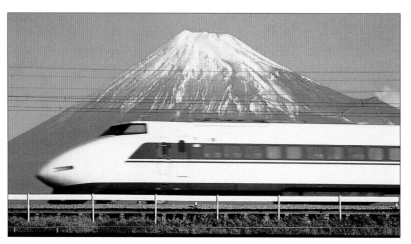

THE BULLET TRAIN
Japan introduced one of the world's first high-speed trains, the bullet, in 1964. Then capable of moving about 130 mph, bullet trains today reach speeds of up to 186 mph. A similarly fast train is being planned for the Washington, D.C., to Boston corridor in the not too distant future.

Safety measures

A fire at King's Cross underground station in 1987 prompted the introduction of a number of new safety measures by London Transport. These included a no-smoking rule in all underground trains and stations. The agency also undertook to remove wooden steps on station escalators and replace them with metal ones.

25 years later came the first authorized use of highway funds for public transportation. More than 13 million Americans now use buses, trains, and subways on a typical weekday, and in the first quarter of 2000, ridership was up almost 5 percent over the same period in 1999.

TRAVEL PATTERNS

During the last quarter of the 20th century, the use of automobiles increased dramatically worldwide and forced a number of developing countries to face many of the same problems of traffic congestion and air pollution that Western countries had been wrestling with for years. Meanwhile, traffic congestion in the industrialized countries also rose at an alarming rate.

Most people are aware that public transportation offers a more environmentally friendly way of traveling, but many of them still prefer to use their cars. Some factors that disincline people to use public transportation include the increased time it often takes, the infrequency of service, and the inadequacy of routes covered. The majority of rural areas tend to be serviced especially poorly, leaving many less populated regions hard to reach by public transportation. Another major concern about using public transportation, primarily in large cities, is fear for personal safety.

Solutions for public transportation

Numerous surveys have been undertaken to establish measures that will improve public transportation and make it more pleasant to use. As a result, some rail networks have introduced schemes to reduce vandalism, assaults, and muggings in or near stations. These include improving station design and

lighting, adding to surveillance on platforms, and increasing the frequency of late-night services.

Some communities have reintroduced once defunct transportation options, such as ferryboat and commuter rail services. Van pools, in which 8 to 10 people working for the same company or in the same office building travel by van, have become a popular way to get to work. Some other innovations include light railways and trolleybuses.

Automobile use could be reduced even further if train and bus companies serving rural and suburban areas would implement initiatives for improving the reliability of services. Little-used routes might easily become more popular if steps were taken to improve the speed, frequency, and comfort of their services. Only a comprehensive network adequately catering to the whole country will persuade people living in or traveling to areas outside urban settings to use public transportation instead of a car.

Providing viable alternatives to the automobile does take investment and planning, but many cities have succeeded in doing just this. Singapore, Tokyo, and Hong Kong, for example, have all developed high-quality integrated transportation systems that are frequent, reliable, and comfortable. Indeed, about two-thirds of all trips in Singapore are now made on the city's public transportation system, which comprises a comprehensive bus network and a Mass Rapid Transit (MRT) railway system, with both aboveground and underground branches. Singapore and Hong Kong have also imposed high annual registration fees and road taxes to make car ownership expensive and therefore less attractive.

Several European cities have also taken steps in recent years to improve their transportation systems. Trams in the German city of Karlsruhe have been adapted so that they can be used on railway lines, meaning that passengers now have no need to change from tram to train. Commuting to work has been reduced by an average of 15 minutes.

Bologna, Italy, has signed up for the International Council for Local Environmental Initiatives Urban CO_2 Reduction Project, which aims to combine green initiatives with a general cleaning up of the transportation system, providing a well-planned, affordable, smooth-running travel option that is also environmentally friendly.

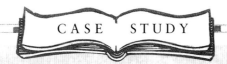
An Anxious Commuter

Many people find commuting on public transportation one of the most stressful aspects of their working day. Crowded conditions and standing for long periods can at best be trying and at worst induce feelings of claustrophobia, but there are ways to overcome these stresses in order to benefit from the positive aspects of public transportation.

Stella is a 40-year-old manager of a beauty salon in the center of a large city. She does not work excessively long hours but is on her feet a lot and often has to work on Saturdays. She travels to work by bus, always at peak hours, and because the bus is usually full when it gets to her stop, she rarely gets a seat. Stella often finds it hard to take a deep breath when she is on the bus and feels hot, sweaty, and giddy, as if she were going to faint. Recently, she has also had pains in her chest and worries that she is going to have a heart attack. Her doctor has assured her that her heart is normal and healthy. He told her that her symptoms are classic signs of a panic attack and are probably brought on by stress.

WHAT SHOULD STELLA DO?

Stella cannot change her job or hours, and the distance to work is too far to walk or bicycle, so she must find ways of coping with the situation. A friend recommended that she see a hypnotherapist to help overcome her anxiety. Learning some relaxation and visualization techniques would help her cope with the crowded conditions on her commuter bus as well. Stella should also exercise regularly to counter the excessive hormones her panic attacks are releasing in her body and to strengthen her leg muscles for the long hours of standing. When she has to work long hours, she should take regular breaks and spend plenty of time relaxing after leaving the salon.

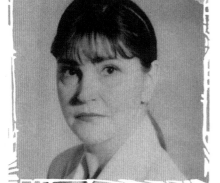

STRESS
External factors that cannot be controlled, such as commuting during rush hour, can result in excess stress.

LIFESTYLE
A tiring workday combined with a long or stressful journey home can cause health problems.

EMOTIONAL HEALTH
Health problems for which a physical cause is not immediately apparent can also cause emotional distress.

Action Plan

LIFESTYLE
Take regular breaks during the day and spend some time in the evenings doing activities that release stress.

EMOTIONAL HEALTH
Visit doctor for regular checkups to be sure that nothing is physically wrong. Practice relaxation techniques until it becomes easy to calm down in stressful situations.

STRESS
Realize that there is no way to avoid the crowds and therefore learn how to cope with them.

HOW THINGS TURNED OUT FOR STELLA

Stella went to see a hypnotherapist, who helped her to develop some relaxation strategies for coping with stress on the bus. She learned controlled deep-breathing techniques, as well as ways to use visualization, and she has found these really help her to keep calm. She also started attending an aerobics class twice a week, which helps her to unwind at the end of the day and recharges her energy levels.

This involves the introduction of new ecologically sound trams and buses, real-time public information at bus stops, promotion of public transportation passes, bicycle rentals within certain areas, and analysis of Car-Free City experiments in Germany.

PUBLIC TRANSPORTATION FOR THE DISABLED AND ELDERLY

Disabled and elderly passengers tend to suffer the most from poor transportation systems because they often have no other way of getting around town. Their mobility and access to vital services in the community are greatly reduced if only a limited number of buses and trains are available. This situation can be damaging to their health and well-being.

At the forefront of current measures to provide better transportation services for the elderly and disabled is the kneeling bus, which can be lowered at the door so that it is level with the pavement, thus allowing easier access for the elderly and persons with physical limitations. Kneeling buses are increasingly available in towns all over the United States. Early indications show that in addition to being more convenient, they are safer than ordinary buses because they make it easier for all passengers to alight.

The Americans with Disabilities Act of 1990 mandated that all new buses and railway and subway cars have lifts or other ways to accommodate wheelchair users. Many local authorities also provide subsidized public transportation for seniors and the disabled, including specially equipped vans.

THE KNEELING BUS
Buses have been designed specifically with the level of the entrance and exit at nearly the same height as the pavement or with the capability of being lowered to this level at bus stops. This helps the elderly, the disabled, and people with children to get on and off the bus more safely and easily.

PUBLIC TRANSPORTATION AND YOUR HEALTH

Using public transportation is healthier than sitting in a car for long periods in heavy traffic, which not only subjects you to traffic fumes but also involves no form of physical activity. Lack of exercise is a problem for about 60 percent of men and women in America. Health organizations around the world, as well as the surgeon general of the United States, emphasize the importance of having a minimum of three 30-minute sessions of exercise each week. Brisk walking for this period of time—for example, to and from a train station or bus stop—could provide baseline protection against the problems associated with lack of exercise.

Older people in particular need a regular regimen of rhythmic, weight-bearing exercise in order to protect bone mineral density against osteoporosis and to maintain the integrity of muscle function. Regular exercise also gives the elderly the physical confidence and ability necessary to avoid falls and consequent hip fractures.

Using public transportation can be mildly demanding on the body. Simply standing on a moving bus or train requires some form of muscle strength to keep your balance. Public transportation also offers the opportunity for exercise in some other, not so obvious ways; for example, you can walk up and down the stairs or escalators to the train platforms or get off the bus one stop early and walk the rest of the way to your destination. This small, regular amount of exercise, carried out as part of a daily routine, can help reduce the risks of hypertension, heart disease, and stroke and make you feel fit and healthy. With a small amount of effort, you can easily include this mild form of exercise in your life.

The health effects of the mental stress and physical inactivity of driving a car have not as yet been quantified. However, driving has no benefits, especially if it replaces exercise, and it definitely pollutes the air and causes environmental damage.

BENEFITS OF CYCLING AND WALKING

Cycling and walking are very effective and inexpensive modes of transportation that do not pollute the environment and keep you fit at the same time. They were once the main methods of getting around—indeed, they still are in many places, such as

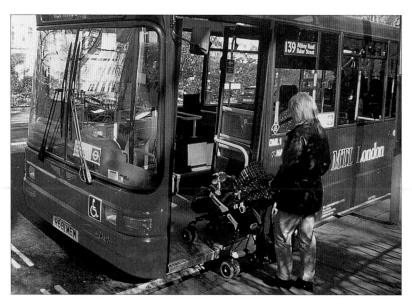

ADJUSTING YOUR BICYCLE TO SUIT YOU

The frame of your bicycle should fit your size and shape. A bicycle salesperson can help you to choose a bike with the correct frame size and adjust your seat and handlebars suitably. There are some principles to follow that can help you make the right choice.

FRAME SIZE
The frame is measured from the center of the bar that runs from the pedals up to the seat and along to the center of the cross-bar. To find the perfect frame size, this measurement should be 14 inches less than your inside leg measurement.

The distance between the seat and the handlebars should be the same as the distance between your fingertips and elbow.

A diamond-framed bike (with a crossbar) has a stronger, lighter frame than an open-framed bike.

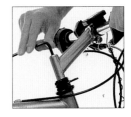

HANDLEBAR HEIGHT
Handlebars should be no higher than the seat to ensure that weight is evenly distributed.

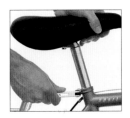

SEAT HEIGHT
Adjust the seat so your knees are slightly bent when your feet are on the pedals.

China—but in general, bicycling and walking have been replaced by the automobile for all but the shortest distances.

The increased use of the car has meant that cyclists today often have to cope with traffic congestion and other hazardous road conditions. Despite recent increases in sales and rentals of bicycles, they still account for only a small percentage of all journeys to work or appointments. Most are kept primarily for use during leisure time.

Many people could easily use a bicycle instead of a car to get to work or appointments. It is estimated that 72 percent of all car trips are under five miles, and this is a comfortable distance for most people to cycle. With a small amount of planning, a bicycle can easily become a viable and enjoyable form of transportation for many more persons.

BENEFITS OF BICYCLING

High pollution levels and the risk of accidents play a significant role in dissuading cyclists from using major roads. However, the associated risks of cycling versus the health benefits suggest that cycling remains a healthy activity worth promoting. Studies that have examined the health risks and health benefits of cycling found that an

CHECKLIST
Cycling is a very healthy way of getting around, but you must be aware of other traffic and observe safety precautions.

✔ *Avoid busy roads and congested traffic as much as possible, especially if you suffer from heart or chest problems.*

✔ *Use bicycle lanes and safe cycling routes whenever possible.*

✔ *Wear a helmet at all times.*

✔ *Always wear bright clothing or reflectors, even during the day.*

✔ *Be sure to clearly signal all your maneuvers.*

✔ *Make sure your bike is road-worthy, with good brakes and a light.*

increase in cycling was particularly beneficial in reducing such health problems as coronary heart disease, obesity, and hypertension, as well as increasing overall fitness. Even in a difficult traffic environment, the benefits gained from regular cycling are likely to outweigh the chances of injury because of cycling accidents.

Cycling to work on a daily basis can produce the health benefits of a specific training program or workout. A recent study of factory workers found that those who cycled to work every day enjoyed a fitness level equivalent to that of individuals 10 years younger; another study found that those who cycled 60 miles a week had an average life expectancy two years longer than that of the general population.

Pollution is cited as a major reason for people not using their bicycles; however, studies have found that the effect of air pollution is actually worse for car drivers and passengers than for cyclists, pedestrians, or bus passengers. This is because polluted air accumulates and produces a tunnel of pollution around the car.

There are economic benefits too. The cost of using a bicycle for a year is only about $120, whereas the expense of owning and operating a car is about $5,200. Walking costs nothing, except for a small investment in a good pair of shoes. And there is plenty of evidence to support the thesis that the health gains from bicycling and walking—both in terms of exercise and reduced air pollution—would save millions in health care costs in the long term.

About 40 percent of automobile trips are less than two miles—a 10-minute bike ride or a 30-minute walk—and these shorter trips are far more polluting on a per mile basis than longer ones. Some 60 percent of the pollution created by an automobile happens in the first few minutes of operation, before pollution control devices can work effectively. According to the World Watch Institute, a 2-mile trip by bicycle would keep about 15 pounds of pollutants out of the air we breathe.

Transporting groceries has always presented a problem for cyclists, but imaginative approaches are being developed to overcome the problem. In 1998 a supermarket chain in Great Britain initiated a pilot program in which a specially designed two-wheel trailer that attaches to any bicycle can be acquired by a shopper at the checkout counter with a small deposit. The trailer must be returned within three days, preferably full of items for recycling. The aim is to encourage more shoppers to consider a bicycle as a practical mode of carrying purchases.

PROMOTING CYCLING

Many European countries have introduced policies that have helped to create a good network of bicycle lanes and safe places to cross busy roads. Some European cities, such as Graz in Austria and Munich in Germany, have seen substantial increases in bicycle use over the past 20 years.

The introduction of bicycle lanes in many American communities has made it easier and safer for bicyclists to get around urban areas. And more funds are now being set aside for such programs. Thanks to the passage of the Intermodal Surface Transportation Efficiency Act in 1992, hundreds of millions of dollars are now being spent annually on development of bicycle and pedestrian facilities, and millions more are being allocated to promoting their use and safety. In addition, many health, park, and education departments are also spending part of their budgets on projects related to bicycle and pedestrian activities.

Other initiatives to encourage people to use their bicycles include increasing the number of secure areas in which to leave bicycles, especially near railway stations and supermarkets. Many business and college campuses are also providing bicycle storage areas (sometimes showers as well) to promote bicycle use for commuting.

Cycling and walking will not only help combat pollution but also improve the health of the public. However, if there are to be significant health benefits to the nation, the government will have to give the same consideration to cyclists and pedestrians that is now given to vehicle drivers.

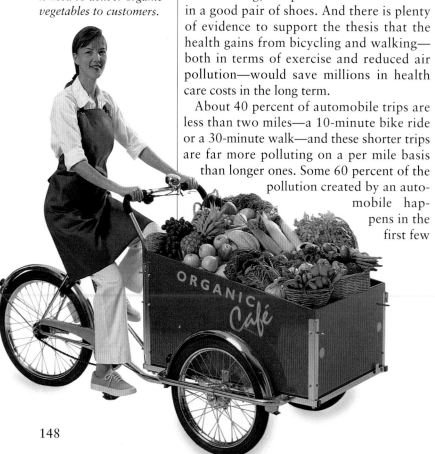

BICYCLE DELIVERIES
Bicycles are convenient for door-to-door deliveries. Bicycle couriers can move around cities faster and less expensively than cars. This tricycle, with a large basket in front, is used to deliver organic vegetables to customers.

AIR TRAVEL

Air travel today is as commonplace as a journey by rail or bus once was. However, people can experience discomfort while flying and feel jet lag after a long trip; remedies are available.

Flying has made traveling the world far faster and easier than it once was. An executive can do business in Seattle today and Tokyo tomorrow, and parents can regularly visit grown children a continent away. But zooming through time zones can have unpleasant effects on the body.

PHYSIOLOGICAL EFFECTS OF AIR TRAVEL

The earth's atmosphere extends about 60 miles above the planet's surface. At sea level the pressure of the air is approximately 1,000 millibars (mb), with some variation according to weather conditions and the time of year. Air pressure diminishes the higher you go above sea level, and though the percentage of oxygen in the air remains constant, less oxygen enters the bloodstream through the lungs. To compensate, the heart and lungs work harder and the body gives off more carbon dioxide, which can upset the biochemical balance in the body. This can result in dizziness, headache, fatigue, nausea, rapid heartbeat, and breathlessness. If fluid builds up in the brain or lungs, a person may also exhibit an unsteady gait, impaired memory and judgment, or blueness of the earlobes, lips, and nail beds.

Cabin pressure on a passenger aircraft flying up to 39,000 feet is usually equivalent to the atmospheric pressure at an altitude of about 6,000 feet. The majority of people are unaffected by this altitude, but a few may experience the symptoms of hypoxia, or insufficient oxygen, mentioned above; these symptoms can usually be cleared up by the administration of oxygen.

Travelers at risk of suffering from a lack of oxygen include those with severe cardiovascular or respiratory problems, a neurological disorder such as a recent stroke or epilepsy, or severe anemia. If you have any of these conditions, you may be advised not to fly. If you are unsure, you should seek medical advice before you travel. If you do have a medical condition and think you might need help boarding the airplane or require oxygen during the flight, notify the airline prior to the departure date.

Carbon monoxide in cigarette smoke reduces the oxygen-carrying ability of the blood, so heavy smokers may also be at risk of discomfort or hypoxia when flying. Smoking is not allowed on any domestic flights in the United States, and several carriers also prohibit it on international trips. This is a step toward making the artificial atmosphere of an airplane cabin healthier and more comfortable for all passengers.

If you are pregnant, you should not fly if you are more than 34 to 36 weeks into the pregnancy. This is because aircraft are not equipped for dealing with an early onset of labor and there is also a risk of fetal hypoxia (insufficient oxygen reaching the baby). For the same reason babies less than 48 hours old should not fly because their lungs are not fully expanded and they may not be able to cope with a low oxygen level.

Changes in air pressure prompt gases in body cavities, such as the inner ear and gut, to expand in volume by about a third. This is what causes popping in the ears on take-off and landing and abdominal bloating and foot swelling during the flight. (Moving

FLIGHT ESSENTIALS
A few provisions can make your flight more comfortable: water to prevent dehydration, earplugs and eyeshades to aid sleep, toothbrush and toothpaste to freshen up before arrival, hand and face moisturizer to prevent dry skin, and candies to suck to prevent your ears from popping.

ADVANCE PREPARATION

It is worth taking a little time to make sure your needs will be covered on a flight.

If you require special food—to meet the requirements of a vegetarian or kosher diet, for example—you should notify the airline at least 24 hours before departure. In fact, you can put in your request when you make your reservation.

If you have a child who will be flying alone, you should ask the airline about its policy concerning unaccompanied minors. Prepare a bag for the child to take along, containing drawing materials, games, books, and little snacks, and include written instructions about who will meet him or her at the destination, along with phone numbers for that person and yourself in case the flight should be delayed.

If you need a wheelchair to board the plane, arrange for that ahead of time also.

around the plane and doing exercises in your seat can help maintain good blood circulation and relieve foot swelling as well.) Carbonated drinks, alcohol, and gas-producing foods such as beans can exacerbate this problem. During a flight, avoid any foods that you know will give you gas, drink plenty of water or fruit juice, and wear loose clothing and comfortable footwear.

Anyone who has ear or sinus problems, a cold, or the flu may find the condition is worse when flying. Taking a decongestant a couple of hours before takeoff can offer some relief and combat pain. Sucking a hard candy, swallowing, and yawning can also provide relief by helping to equalize pressure on both sides of the eardrum. Giving babies a bottle during ascent and descent will alleviate ear pain, as will allowing them to cry, although other passengers may not appreciate the latter. People who have had a recent middle ear infection should wait until the eardrum has healed properly. Following inner ear surgery you should wait at least two weeks before traveling.

If you are going on a diving vacation, allow at least 24 hours between flying and diving. The pressure under water is much denser than that in the air, and the massive contrast between the two may lead to a potentially fatal condition known as decompression sickness, or the bends. Symptoms include headache, pain in the arms, legs, and joints, choking or vomiting, and in rare cases, paralysis or circulatory collapse.

If you have recently had abdominal or chest surgery, pneumothorax (collapsed lung), or gastrointestinal bleeding, you should seek advice from your doctor before getting on an airplane. The pressure changes may cause severe complications. Other unforeseen problems may also occur. For example, if you are wearing a plaster cast, you may have to have it split because air trapped under the cast can expand and compress the limb. Also, any swelling you have may worsen during air travel, and a cast may become too tight and constrict the limb.

Dehydration
During a flight dehydration can be a problem because the cabin air is very dry. The condition can be prevented by drinking plenty of water or fruit juice. Alcohol and caffeinated beverages should be avoided or kept to a minimum because they are diuretics and make dehydration worse. Using a moisturizer can help to keep your skin from feeling taut and dry. It is advisable to remove contact lenses before flying because your eyes will become drier, which can make your lenses uncomfortable and could even harm your corneas.

Swelling
If you are in an airplane for a long time, the prolonged sitting combined with the low air pressure can make your feet and ankles swell. This is why shoes feel tight at the end of a flight. To make yourself more comfortable, wear sensible shoes, preferably with laces so the fit can be loosened, or remove them during the flight. Keeping both your feet slightly raised above the floor on the special footrests provided or on your hand luggage can help alleviate discomfort. If possible, take a walk around the cabin every hour or so to exercise your feet. You can also perform various foot and lower leg exercises while seated (see opposite page). This will improve blood circulation to your limbs and also reduce the risk of a blood clot developing in the lower leg—a very rare condition but one that could lead to a pulmonary embolism in the lungs. Taking in lots of fluids to avoid becoming dehydrated also reduces the risk of blood clots.

Motion sickness
Nausea, vomiting, and sweating triggered by motion are caused by a disturbance of the balance center in the inner ear, which is closely linked by nerves to the brain's vomiting center. The symptoms can be made

worse by anxiety, fumes, poor ventilation, and looking at a horizon that appears out of sync with your sense of balance. To cope better with travel sickness, avoid alcohol, fatty foods, and large meals, but make sure that your stomach is not empty; eat a light meal or snack before you travel.

Some people find that elasticized bands that press on an acupressure point on the inner wrists offer relief. Certain medications, including scopolamine (administered by a skin patch) and antihistamines like Dramamine, can help prevent motion sickness. These need to be taken before you embark on your trip. You should be aware that some travel sickness drugs cause drowsiness, so don't plan on driving right after you arrive at your destination. One of the best natural remedies for motion sickness is ginger, which can be taken as a tea, capsules, or tablets, or in its candied form. It has no side effects.

JET LAG

The human body is governed by rhythms of sleep and wakefulness known as circadian rhythms. These work on a 24-hour basis, prompting us to feel sleepy at night and to wake up in the morning. They are influenced by various environmental factors, including daylight and darkness, time and temperature, and also social activities, such as mealtimes and work. Jet lag occurs when we travel to a different time zone, which puts the body out of sync with our local time. It is a modern phenomenon caused entirely by air travel. For previous generations travel was slow enough for the body to adjust gradually.

Although there are things you can do to help prevent and recover from jet lag, there is no instant remedy. Jet lag results from stress to your body's biological clock, and you must allow your body time to adjust. The best thing you can do is make sure you are fit and healthy before you fly.

Jet lag can manifest itself as fatigue, insomnia, anxiety, loss of appetite, and diminished ability to concentrate. Symptoms generally occur most noticeably when you cross at least three time zones. It is also thought to take longer to adjust to travel eastward than westward because you are creating an artificially short day. This means that when it is time to go to bed, you are not ready to sleep. Symptoms do not usually last for more than three days.

Children may take longer than adults to adjust to the difference, so parents should be prepared for disturbed nights on arrival.

Managing jet lag

Although there is no instant cure for jet lag, many steps can be taken to reduce its effects. Frequent travelers often formulate their own regimens to combat the effects suffered after crossing several time zones.

Some of the problems associated with jet lag can be minimized with advance planning. Adjust your watch to the new time zone as soon as possible so you are mentally prepared. A morning departure for eastward flights with an afternoon or early evening arrival is ideal because it gives you the chance to have a light meal and some time for relaxation before bedtime. More

IN-FLIGHT FOOT CARE

The low air pressure in airplanes prompts gases in the body cavities to expand, which makes the feet swell and slows the circulation. Wearing slippers in flight is more comfortable, and moving your feet regularly keeps the blood circulating. Here are some simple exercises that can be done at your seat.

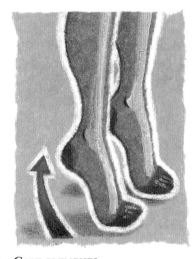

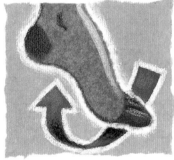

FOOT CIRCLES
Lift your foot off the ground and slowly rotate it in each direction. Repeat with the other foot.

CALF CLENCHES
With both of your feet on the floor, slowly raise your legs onto your tiptoes and tighten the calf muscles. Hold for about 5 seconds. Repeat several times.

FOOT MASSAGE
Grip the sole of your foot with your fingers and massage the top of the foot with your thumbs, using a slow circular motion.

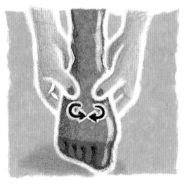

MEAL PLANNING TO REDUCE JET LAG

Jet lag results from the body clock being disturbed by traveling across time zones. Some nutritionists believe that the fatigue and sluggishness can be reduced by adjusting what you eat on the day before flying and by avoiding alcohol, caffeine, and rich, fatty foods during the flight. One approach is to make the first two meals on the day before flying rich in proteins—for example, milk, yogurt, cheese, fish, and meat—and the final meal rich in carbohydrates, such as pasta, rice, potatoes, and bread, plus vegetables or a light salad. Some people find that they feel better if they eat lightly—for instance, having broth, fruit, a light salad, and toast—the day before a long flight and follow the meal pattern given here upon arrival.

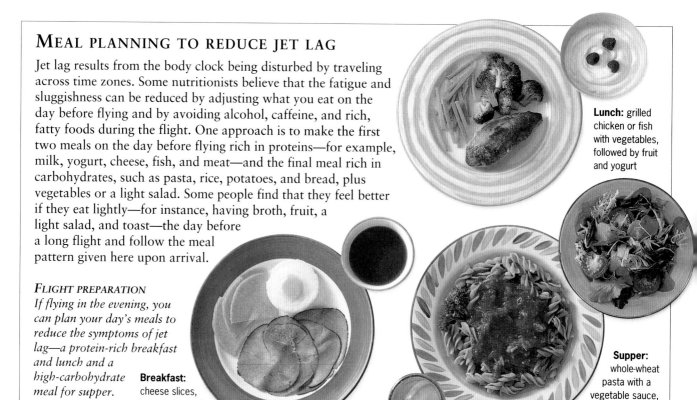

Lunch: grilled chicken or fish with vegetables, followed by fruit and yogurt

Supper: whole-wheat pasta with a vegetable sauce, plus salad and a glass of water

FLIGHT PREPARATION
If flying in the evening, you can plan your day's meals to reduce the symptoms of jet lag—a protein-rich breakfast and lunch and a high-carbohydrate meal for supper.

Breakfast: cheese slices, ham, eggs, and herbal tea

Sleep aids

It is best to use a natural sleep aid, such as milk or chamomile tea, to promote sleep during a flight or for a night or two at your destination. Some sleeping tablets can slow circulation and cause dehydration during a long flight and leave you feeling fuzzy-headed the next day. Also, you should not drive for at least 24 hours after taking them.

airlines are now scheduling daytime flights, although they are still rare. Your mental and physical ability is also affected by disturbed sleep patterns; if you are traveling on business, try to schedule important meetings at least 24 hours after your arrival to allow time to adjust to your destination time zone. This also applies to the return journey.

All drinks containing caffeine are best avoided during a long flight because they are stimulants that can keep you awake longer. It is best to avoid them also the day before you travel. Dehydration can aggravate the symptoms of jet lag, so make sure you drink plenty of nonalcoholic beverages, such as water, juice, or herbal tea, before and during the flight. Rich and fatty foods should also be avoided throughout the day before you travel because they will make you lethargic and less able to cope with the changes in your circadian rhythms.

Studies have shown that changing your eating patterns before a long trip can alter the brain chemicals that prompt you to sleep and wake up. Various approaches have been suggested. One is to eat protein-rich foods for the two meals before you travel—this would be breakfast and lunch if you have an evening flight—and complex

carbohydrates for the meal on the plane, which will promote relaxation and possibly sleep. When you arrive at your destination, observe local mealtimes to help your body adjust to the new time zone, but follow the meal plan above for the first 24 hours after arrival to maximize energy levels.

Some travelers have had success with a couple of products designed especially for dealing with jet lag. One of them, called the Jet Lag Eliminator, is based on stimulating certain acupressure points to help the body adjust its circadian rhythms from the departure time zone to the destination zone. Another product, called No Jet Lag, is a homeopathic formula. Both products are available at stores that specialize in travel products and at some airport shops.

You can also use essential oils in various combinations to help you sleep or wake up. If you arrive in the evening, adding a couple of drops of chamomile, geranium, or lavender oil to your bathwater can help you wind down before bedtime. Alternatively, rosemary or eucalyptus can energize and wake you up if you have an early morning arrival. A few drops of lavender oil on a handkerchief may also help you to sleep during a nighttime flight.

TRAVEL ABROAD

If an exotic location is your vacation destination, you may need to take some precautions against possible health hazards that can spoil more than just your vacation.

Foreign travel can be both exciting and enlightening, but at the same time it can expose you to illnesses you probably would not encounter in your everyday life at home. There are measures you can take before leaving home and at your destination to avoid infection. Seek advice from your travel agent and doctor before you leave.

TRAVEL-RELATED ILLNESSES

A common ailment that travelers experience in foreign countries is diarrhea. Between 20 and 50 percent of people who travel abroad each year endure a bout that causes them great discomfort. Diarrhea can be caused by a variety of organisms transmitted through food or water. It is usually self-limiting, lasting for one to three days at the most, but it can disrupt your plans greatly. You should take all the precautions you can to prevent getting diarrhea (see page 155).

Malaria, an infectious disease caused by any of four strains of the *Plasmodium* protozoan, is also becoming increasingly common as more people travel to exotic destinations. Symptoms vary according to the strain of

THE SPREAD OF MALARIA

Malaria is a major health problem in the tropics and affects at least 300 million people worldwide each year. The disease is spread by the bites of infected mosquitoes, which release parasites (plasmodia) that invade the liver. These plasmodia redevelop in the blood into other forms that can infect mosquitoes.

MALARIA CYCLE
Malaria is easily passed from mosquito to human and back again, which makes it a difficult disease to control.

An uninfected mosquito bites an infected person, thereby becoming infected itself.

■ **Prevalent malarial areas**

When an infected mosquito bites a human, parasitic organisms, or plasmodia, in the mosquito's saliva enter the bloodstream.

Other plasmodia develop into forms that can infect mosquitoes when they bite humans.

Plasmodia make their way to the liver, where they multiply.

Plasmodia invade the red blood cells and cause them to rupture and release more plasmodia.

plasmodium involved, but they typically include intermittent fever, chills, sweating, achiness, throbbing headache, and a generally ill feeling. Once the fever subsides, the patient usually feels better until the next attack, which may come within 72 hours.

The disease is transmitted by the anopheles mosquito, which is found only in hot and humid areas, including the tropical regions of Africa, South America, India, and Indonesia. Worldwide, an astonishing 300 to 500 million people contract malaria each year, and between 2 and 3 million die as a result. The majority of victims are children who live in tropical Africa.

Alarmingly, malaria is becoming resistant to common antimalarial drugs, such as chloroquine; other medications, such as larium (mefloquine hydrochloride), can cause serious side effects. Nevertheless, you should have antimalarial treatment if you are visiting an infected area and be vigilant against being bitten.

Avoiding mosquito bites

Mosquito bites produce redness, itching, and discomfort because a mosquito injects a histamine into your blood when it bites. Some people are more sensitive than others to this allergic reaction. There are various ways to prevent mosquito bites and thus protect yourself from malaria and any other mosquito-borne infections. One of the best is to apply an insect repellent to your skin every three to four hours—the most effective ones contain diethyltolumide (DEET) or lemon-eucalyptus. In field trials in Tanzania, lemon-eucalyptus was as effective as DEET in repelling mosquitoes, and it is more suitable for children. Some people claim that brewer's yeast tablets or yeast extract products make you less susceptible to insect bites, but this has not been proved.

It is possible to buy clothing that is impregnated with insect repellent; alternatively, you could use wrist and ankle bands that have been treated with repellent—wrists and ankles receive the most bites. Mosquitoes bite mainly between dusk and dawn, so you should cover up after sunset or around dawn by wearing long trousers and a long-sleeved shirt.

The effectiveness of mosquito nets is often underestimated. Those that are sprayed with insecticide, such as permethrin, save the lives of thousands of African children every year. Surveys carried out in 1997 in Africa found that putting nets around children's beds at night reduced the mortality rate by 17 to 33 percent.

Mosquito nets can be easily obtained from travel stores and catalogs. The most effective ones are treated with insecticide, which needs to be reapplied every six months if you are abroad for a long time. You can also spray insecticide under the nets before bedtime and inside the room at dusk to destroy mosquitoes that enter during the day. However, this procedure must be done judiciously to maintain a healthy environment in which to sleep. Insecticide coils or plug-in vaporizers are also effective at repelling the insects.

GENERAL HEALTH PRECAUTIONS

Contaminated food can be the cause of many of the diseases contracted in underdeveloped countries, but there are several ways that you can minimize the risks. First, always make sure that any hot food you eat is thoroughly cooked and served piping hot. It is best to avoid buffet meals because food left at room temperature for a few hours is a suitable breeding ground for bacteria. Be especially wary of eating raw or undercooked meat, and check that fish and shellfish are fresh and come from a reliable source.

Even if the weather is very hot, avoid eating salads and raw vegetables unless you know they have been thoroughly washed using safe water. It is a good idea to peel all fruits and vegetables that are to be eaten raw. You should also avoid drinking unpasteurized cow, sheep, or goat milk. If in

MOSQUITO NETS
Mosquito nets are essential in many tropical countries to ward off insects while sleeping. Ideally, the net should be impregnated with an insecticide, free of holes, and tucked into the mattress all around.

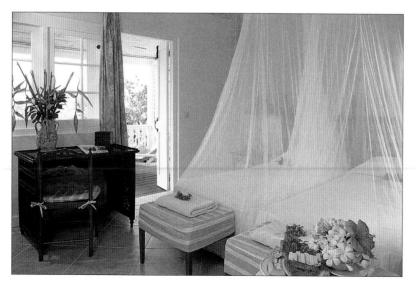

THE DO'S AND DON'TS OF SAFE EATING

Whenever you travel in developing areas, you must be careful about what you eat and drink. There are many ways in which food and water can become contaminated and cause disease. However, a few simple precautions can prevent infection.

DO	DON'T
buy packaged or sealed food.	buy unpackaged food that may have been exposed to flies or other pests.
eat freshly cooked food that is still piping hot.	eat food that has been kept warm, such as on a buffet.
wash everything in clean, purified water.	drink local tap water or have ice in drinks.
peel all fruits and vegetables to be eaten raw.	eat fruits or vegetables raw unless peeled.
check the kitchen in a restaurant for cleanliness.	buy food exposed to traffic pollution at the roadside.
avoid unpasteurized dairy products.	eat ice cream from unreliable sources, such as a kiosk.
drink bottled mineral water and make sure that the seal is intact when you buy it.	eat uncooked shellfish where waters are polluted.

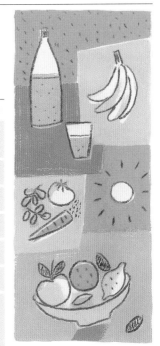

doubt, you can pasteurize milk yourself by bringing it to the boiling point and then allowing it to cool. Stay clear of unpasteurized mik products, such as ice cream and cheese, from an uncertain source.

Avoiding contaminated water

Drinking water is a frequent source of infection in all regions where sanitation systems are poor. Even in cities and towns where water has been fully treated, there can be problems in the distribution. When uncertain about the source of water, you should boil any that you drink to be on the safe side. Alternatively, you can buy a water purifier that contains an iodine resin and a charcoal filter, which will destroy bacteria, viruses, and contamination from parasites and also improve the water's taste and smell. Purifiers with ceramic and membrane filters also work for bacteria but may not destroy viruses. Tablets of chlorine and iodine added to water and then left to stand for about 30 minutes will also disinfect it. Treated water should be stored in the same container it was treated in or in another sterile container to prevent recontamination.

If you are unable to purify water, you should take steps to avoid local tap water. Drink and clean your teeth in bottled water, making sure the seal on the bottle is intact when you buy it. Hot drinks, such as tea and coffee, are safe as long as the milk added is pasteurized, and you can also drink bottled soft drinks and beers, although drinking too many beers is not a good idea because you could become dehydrated. It is best not to add ice to your drinks.

Take care when swimming or bathing in fresh water because it may be contaminated with sewage or even schistosomiasis, a parasitic disease that can cause liver problems. Poorly chlorinated swimming pools may also carry infections such as giardia and hepatitis A. If the swimming pool smells of chlorine, it is usually safe to use, but too much of this chemical can cause respiratory difficulties and skin problems.

If you are vacationing near a coastline, try to ascertain that the local beaches are clean and safe for bathing before you use them. Many coastlines in both industrial and developing nations have become contaminated by litter, sewage, and industrial waste. In 1987 an award called the European Blue Flag was introduced that recognizes clean, well-managed beaches in 19 European countries. To be eligible for a Blue Flag a beach must meet 26 criteria. These include easy and safe access to the beach, regular cleaning and maintenance, a sufficient number of lifeguards and litter bins, and adequate first-aid equipment. The water must be unaffected by industrial waste or sewage and have no signs of gross pollution from oil or human waste.

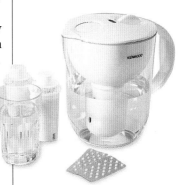

WATER PURIFIERS
To make sure water is safe to drink, use a water filter and sterilize it with special disinfectant tablets, or buy bottled water, checking that the seal is intact.

Ticks

In addition to taking precautions against mosquito bites (see page 154), you should also take care not to be bitten by ticks. These are common in temperate and warm regions, and because of the global climate change, they are now spreading to places where they were previously unknown. There are several types of ticks, but all of them feed on the blood of a host—an animal or a human. They can transmit serious illnesses like Lyme disease and many other conditions. The symptoms of Lyme disease, which you are more likely to get in North America than abroad, are flulike, with a fever, headache, and aching muscles. If not treated, Lyme disease can persist for years.

When visiting areas where ticks are common, wear long trousers tucked into socks and a long-sleeved shirt and check your skin regularly if you are walking or camping in infested areas, paying particular attention to the warm areas of your body, such as the armpits. If you do find a tick, remove it by

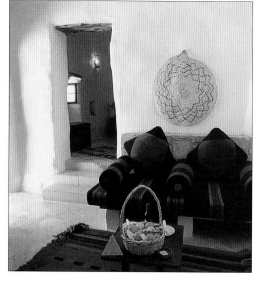

ECO-FRIENDLY TOURIST RESORT
A traditional village in Jordan was converted into this award-winning eco-friendly resort. Rooms are very simply furnished using local materials, and most of the food is grown on-site.

gently rocking it from side to side. If you use tweezers or a tissue to hold it, you reduce the risk of pulling out the tick body and leaving its mouthparts in the skin, which can then become infected.

IMMUNIZATION

In advance of your trip, seek advice from your doctor or the consulate or embassy of each country you plan to visit to find out if you require any vaccinations. A full course of vaccines to ensure maximum protection can take six to eight weeks to complete. The vaccine required depends on your destination, the length of your stay, the time of year, whether you will be sleeping under canvas, the activities planned, and any pre-existing conditions or allergies.

Immunization is a way of building up the body's defense system to resist an infection by introducing a small amount of the organism responsible for that disease. It is a generally safe and effective method for protecting against potentially dangerous diseases. If you are pregnant or think you might be allergic to a particular vaccine, seek your doctor's advice.

Some vaccines are compulsory; several countries require a yellow fever vaccination before you can enter. The most common vaccinations required are for tetanus, hepatitis A, and typhoid. Others are for rabies, meningitis, and Japanese B encephalitis.

THE TRAVELER'S CHECKLIST

Before you embark on a trip, you should check the health risks of your destination; these will depend not only on the countries you may be visiting but also on the time of year and type of vacation. If it is a hot country, sun protection is vital, so pack sunblock, a wide-brimmed hat, and sunglasses. Health insurance is important wherever you travel, but especially in countries where disease is rife or where you are pursuing any risky activities, such as skiing.

ESSENTIALS FOR A SUITCASE
Here are several items you should pack to ensure optimum health and comfort while traveling.

A luggage label attached securely to your suitcase will aid in retrieval should it become lost.

Sunscreens for skin, hair, and lips and aloe vera lotion for sunburn are essential in hot countries.

A broad-brimmed hat will help prevent sunburn and heat stroke when you are traveling in a hot region.

First-aid items should include Band-Aids and safety pins, plus antiseptic cream or comfrey ointment mixed with tea tree oil to cleanse and heal wounds.

Health insurance is often forgotten but is one of the most important items of all.

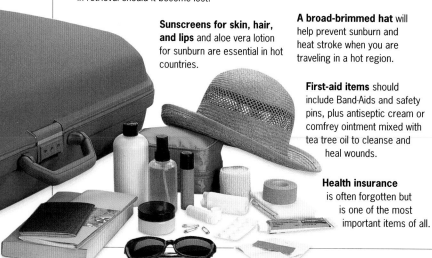

INDEX

ACKNOWLEDGMENTS

Carroll & Brown Limited
would like to thank
Camden and Islington Health
  Authority, London
Kevin Clinton, Royal Society for the
  Prevention of Accidents
Ecological Design Association,
  Great Britain
Gail and Snowdon Architects
London Transport Commission
Lorna Howarth, Editor, *Positive News*
National Radiological Protection
  Board
Helen Pointer, Croydon Eye Hospital
Michael Rose

Editorial assistance
Dawn Henderson

Design assistance
Simon Daley
Carmel O'Neil

Picture research
Richard Soar

Photograph sources
Cover, Goddard Space Flight
  Centre
  6 Carroll & Brown Ltd Photo
     Archive
  8 (Top) Pictor International
     (Bottom) AKG London
  9 Environmental Images/Mark
     Fallander
 10 Ecoscene/Bruce Harber
 11 Ecoscene/Bruce Harber
 13 Robert Harding Picture Library
 14 Telegraph Colour Library
 16 (Top left) Elizabeth Whiting
     Associates, (Top right) Goddard
     Space Flight Centre
 19 (Top) BSIP Martin PL/Science
     Photo Library, (Bottom) Images
     Colour Library
 21 CDC/Science Photo Library
 22 Carroll & Brown Ltd Photo
     Archive
 24 (Top) Graseby Anderson Ltd,
     (Bottom) Hulton Getty
 26 Eye Ubiquitous

 27 Simon Fraser/Science Photo
     Library
 28 Corbis-Bettmann/UPI
 29 (Top) Simon Fraser/Science
     Photo Library, (Bottom) Will &
     Deni McIntyre/Science Photo
     Library
 32 The Image Bank
 36 Angela Hampton, Family Life
     Pictures
 39 Adam Hart-Davis/Science Photo
     Library
 41 Pictor International
 44 Tony Stone Images
 47 Russ Mann/Science Photo Library
 56 CNRI/Science Photo Library
 57 J.C. Revy/Science Photo Library
 58 Rory McClenaghan/Science
     Photo Library
 59 Keeler Ltd
 62 Dr G. Oran/Science Photo
     Library
 63 Images Colour Library
 64 Tony Stone Images
 68 Jonathan Ashton/Science Photo
     Library
 70 Ecoscene/Martin Jones
 71 Ecoscene/Nick Hawkes
 74 Pictor International
 75 Environmental Images/Martin
     Bond
 78 Hulton Getty
 80 Adrian Arbib Photography
 82 Turkish Tourist Board
 83 Pictor International
 84 Eric Crichton (Designer, Roger
     Platt)
 88 Mike Birkhead/Oxford
     Scientific Films
 89 (Top) Harry Smith Collection,
     (Bottom) Carroll & Brown Ltd
     Photo Archive
 90 Derek St Romaine
 92 Ace Photo Library
 99 Elizabeth Whiting Associates/
     Mark Luscombe Whyte
100 IKEA
102 Neil Lorimer/Elizabeth Whiting
     Associates'
107 Elizabeth Whiting Associates/
     Brian Harrison

109 Elizabeth Whiting Associates/
     Tom Leighton
110 Elizabeth Whiting Associates/
     Gary Chowanetz
112 Elizabeth Whiting Associates/
     Rodney Hyett
114 (Top left) Feng Shui Network/
     Harry Archer, (Top right) Ace
     Photo Library, (Bottom right)
     Andrew Southall/Builder Group
115 The Image Bank
116 The Image Bank
120 Ace Photo Library
123 *Feng Shui for Modern Living*
130 Andy Bell/Kyle Karate Club
131 *Shotokan Karate Magazine*
134 Sally & Richard Greenhill Photo
     Library
137 (Top) Dr Linda Stannard, UCT/
     Science Photo Library, (Bottom)
     Tony Stone Images
140 Tony Stone Images
141 Britax Excelsior Ltd
144 Tony Stone Images
146 London Transport Museum
153 (Left) Dr Gopal Murti/Science
     Photo Library, (Bottom) Eye of
     Science/Science Photo Library,
     (Right) Telegraph Colour
     Library
154 Robert Harding Picture Library
156 Mark Edwards/Still Pictures

Illustrators
John Geary
Carol Hill
Sally Kindberg
Natasha Stewart
Paul Williams
Angela Wood

Photographic assistance
Colin Tatham

Hair and make-up
Bettina Graham
Kim Menzies

075–016–01